RENAL DIET COOKBOOK

FOR BEGINNERS

A Step-by-Step Guide to Understanding Kidneys, Kidney Diseases and Treatment Procedures, Complete with the Best Kidney-Friendly Recipes for Beginners

Sophia Parks

© **Copyright 2020 by (Sophia Parks)- All rights reserved.**

This document is geared towards providing exact and reliable information in regards to the topic and issue covered. The publication is sold with the idea that the publisher is not required to render accounting, officially permitted, or otherwise, qualified services. If advice is necessary, legal or professional, a practiced individual in the profession should be ordered.

From a Declaration of Principles which was accepted and approved equally by a Committee of the American Bar Association and a Committee of Publishers and Associations.

In no way is it legal to reproduce, duplicate, or transmit any part of this document in either electronic means or in printed format. Recording of this publication is strictly prohibited and any storage of this document is not allowed unless with written permission from the publisher. All rights reserved.

The information provided herein is stated to be truthful and consistent, in that any liability, in terms of inattention or otherwise, by any usage or abuse of any policies, processes, or directions contained within is the solitary and utter responsibility of the recipient reader. Under no circumstances will any legal responsibility or blame be held against the publisher for any reparation, damages, or monetary loss due to the information herein, either directly or indirectly.

Respective authors own all copyrights not held by the publisher.

The information herein is offered for informational purposes solely, and is universal as so. The presentation of the information is without contract or any type of guarantee assurance.

The trademarks that are used are without any consent, and the publication of the trademark is without permission or backing by the trademark owner. All trademarks and brands within this book are for clarifying purposes only and are the owned by the owners themselves, not affiliated with this document.

Table of Contents

Chapter 1- Introduction 7

Chapter 2- Treating Kidney Disease 11

Chapter 3- Dialysis and Problems 21

Chapter 4- Diet 24

Chapter 5- Frequently Asked Questions 31

Breakfasts 36

    1. Herbed Omelet 36

    2. Fruit Omelet 37

    3. Old Fashioned Pancakes 38

    4. French Toast 39

    5. Corn Pudding 39

    6. Kale and Cheddar Frittata 40

    7. Spanish Tortilla or Omelet 41

    8. Egg Salad on Homemade Biscuit 43

    9. Apple and Zucchini Harvest Muffins 46

    10. Banana Chocolate Chip Muffins 47

First Course 49

    11. Curry Chicken 49

    12. Spicy Lamb 50

    13. Special Pizza 51

    14. Slow-Cooked Lemon Chicken 52

    15. Classic Beef Stroganoff with Egg Noodles 54

    16. Roast Pork Loin with Sweet and Tart Apple Stuffing 55

    17. Slow-Cooked Bavarian Pot Roast 57

    18. Herb-Roasted Chicken Breasts 58

    19. Roasted Turkey 59

    20. Ratatouille 61

Seafood 63

    21. Baked fish 63

22. Supreme of Seafood 64

23. Tuna-Noodle Skillet Dinner 65

24. Crab-Stuffed shrimp 66

25. Tuna Veggie Salad 67

26. Cilantro-Lime Cod 69

27. Grilled Trout 69

28. Crunchy Oven-Fried Catfish 70

29. Linguine with Garlic and Shrimp 71

30. Jambalaya 73

Poultry 75

31. Turkey & Noodles 75

32. Barbecue Cups 76

33. Crispy Oven Fried Chicken 77

34. Jalepeno Pepper Chicken 78

35. Stuffed Green Peppers 79

36. Easy Chicken and Pasta Dinner 80

37. Chicken Nuggets with Honey Mustard Dipping Sauce 81

38. Indian Chicken Curry 82

39. Chicken and Summer Vegetable Kebabs 83

40. Easy Turkey Sloppy Joes 84

Meat 86

41. Chili Rice with Beef 86

42. Parsley Burger 87

43. Swedish Meatballs 88

44. Open-Faced Steak & Onion Sandwich 89

45. Homemade Pan Sausage 90

46. Spicy Beef Stir-Fry 91

47. Pasta with Cheesy Meat Sauce 92

48. Hawaiian-Style Slow-Cooked Pulled Pork 93

Vegetables 95

49. Coleslaw 95

50. Vegetables & Rice 96

51. Favorite Green Beans 97

52. Roasted Red Pepper with Basil, Vegan Provolone Cheese Sandwiches 98

53. Vegetarian Egg Fried Rice 99

54. Spicy Chickpeas (Chana Masala) 100

55. Breakfast Burrito 101

56. Garlicky Penne Pasta with Asparagus 102

57. Vegetarian Pizza 103

58. Tempeh Pita Sandwiches 104

59. Veggie Strata 105

60. Fresh Tofu Spring Rolls 107

Stews 109

61. Chicken Stew 109

62. Beef Casserole 110

63. Beef Stew with Carrots and Mushrooms 111

64. Beef Barley Stew 113

65. Chicken and White Bean Chili Stew 114

66. Chicken Pot Pie Stew 115

67. Kidney-Friendly Navy Bean Stew 117

Soups 119

68. Beef & Vegetable Soup 119

69. Chicken Noodle Soup 120

70. Turkey, Wild Rice, and Mushroom Soup 121

71. Cream of Chicken Wild Rice Asparagus Soup 122

72. Spring Vegetable Soup 124

73. Homemade Kidney-Friendly Cream of Mushroom Soup 125

74. Rotisserie Chicken Noodle Soup 126

75. Beef and Cabbage Vegetable Soup 127

76. Five Ingredient Vegetable Broth 128

77. Hearty Vegetable Soup 128

78. Lower Potassium Potato Soup 129

79. Carrot Ginger Soup 130

Smoothies and Juices 132

80. Chocolate Smoothie 132

81. Watermelon Bliss 133

82. Cran-tastic 133

83. Bahama Breeze 134

84. Very Berry Goodness 135

85. What a Peach 136

- *86. Blueberry Blast Smoothie* ... 136
- *87. Easy Pineapple Protein Smoothie* ... 137
- *88. Mixed Berry Protein Smoothie* ... 138
- *89. Kidney Nourishing Smoothie* ... 138
- *90. Four Ingredient Simple Blueberry Smoothie* ... 139
- *91. Watermelon Summer Cooler* ... 140
- *92. Lemonade* ... 141

Desserts ... 142

- *93. Scarlet Frozen Fantasy* ... 142
- *94. Baked Egg Custard* ... 143
- *95. Pineapple Pudding* ... 144
- *96. Old Fashioned Pound Cake* ... 145
- *97. Carrot Cake* ... 146
- *98. Pumpkin Strudel* ... 147
- *99. Sunburst Lemon Bars* ... 149
- *100. Fruit in The Clouds* ... 150

Conclusion ... 152

Chapter 1- Introduction

The kidneys are two organs that are shaped like beans, both around the size of a tennis ball. They are situated on either side of your spine, just under the rib cage.

Approximately half a cup of blood is recycled each minute by healthy kidneys, extracting waste, and excess water to produce urine. Via two small muscular tubes called ureters, one on either side of the bladder, the urine goes from the kidneys to the urinary bladder. The urine is stored in the bladder. The urinary tract includes the kidneys, bladder, and ureters.

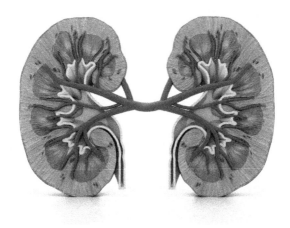

What is the importance of kidneys?

Your kidneys expel your body's waste products and excess fluids. Your kidneys also expel acid made by your cells and maintain the number of salts, water, and minerals such as calcium, phosphorus, potassium, and sodium in your bloodstream.

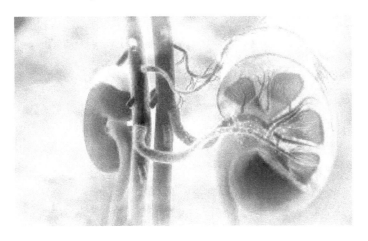

Muscles, nerves, and other tissues in the body cannot function normally without this stability.

The kidneys also generate substances that control blood pressure.

They make blood cells.

How do kidneys operate?

Millions of filtering units termed nephrons make up one of the kidneys. A filter named the glomerulus and a tubule is included in any nephron. The nephrons function in a 2-step process: the glomerulus filters the blood, and the tubule returns the appropriate substances to the bloodstream and eliminates waste.

Each nephron has a blood-filtering glomerulus and a tubule that restores the appropriate substances to your blood and removes excess waste. Waste and extra water are converted into urine.

Blood is filtered by the glomerulus. As blood ran into nephrons, it joins an array of small blood vessels the glomerulus. The glomerulus's thin structure causes small particles, waste, and fluid to flow into the tubule, mainly water. The blood vessel retains bigger molecules, such as blood cells and proteins.

The tubule returns useful substances and removes wastes.

A blood vessel flows with the tubule. The blood vessel helps to reabsorb almost all the water and minerals the body requires, while the diluted fluid travels along the tubule. The tubule enables the blood to expel extra acid. The leftover waste and fluid are urine.

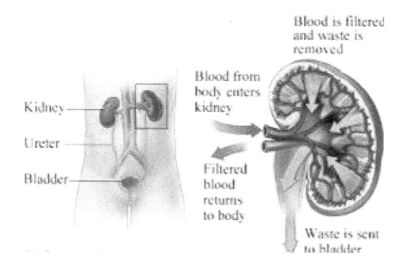

What's kidney disease?

Kidney disease may affect the body's functionality to purify the blood, filter excess fluids from your bloodstream, and control blood pressure. It may also impact the formation of red blood cells and the required synthesis of vitamin D for bone protection.

Waste materials and fluid will build up in your body if your kidneys are harmed. This can cause ankle swelling, fatigue, exhaustion, inadequate sleep, and breathlessness. The harm will get worse without medication, and your kidneys can eventually stop functioning. This is serious, and it can be very dangerous.

Causes of kidney disease

Acute Kidney Disease: Experts call it acute kidney damage or acute renal failure if the kidneys unexpectedly stop functioning. The key reasons are:

- Not adequate blood supply to the kidneys
- Direct injury to your kidneys
- Backed up urine in the kidneys
- Such incidents may occur when you:
- Get a severe blood loss accident, such as in a traffic accident,
- Your muscle tissue starts to break down or is dehydrated, sending extra protein into the blood.
- You go into shock because of a harmful illness called sepsis.
- Have a big prostate which blocks the flow of your urine.
- Take some medications or have been around toxins that specifically affect the kidney.
- Have complications such as preeclampsia and eclampsia during pregnancy.
- Autoimmune disorders can also cause acute kidney damage as the immune system damages the body.

- Individuals with the serious cardiac or liver disease typically often suffer acute kidney damage.

Who can get CKD?

- High-risk individuals include people with hypertension, diabetes, or a family history of kidney disease.
- Hispanics, African Americans, American Indians, Pacific Islanders, and senior citizens are at higher risk.

The Symptoms

Many individuals might not get severe symptoms until their renal disease has progressed. You may see, however, that you:

- Feeling drained and getting less energy
- Getting problems focusing
- Getting a low appetite
- Had problems sleeping
- Muscle cramping in the evening
- Getting bloated feet and ankles
- Have puffiness, particularly in the morning, near your eyes
- Have itchy, dry skin
- Urinating more frequently, particularly at night

Chapter2- Treating Kidney Disease

Treatment for kidney disease is dictated by the problem's source and extent. Treating the chronic health condition will delay kidney disease development. Your doctors will use one or even more techniques to track your health if your kidneys start to lose their work gradually. Your doctor will help you preserve the operation of your kidneys for as long as possible by monitoring you carefully.

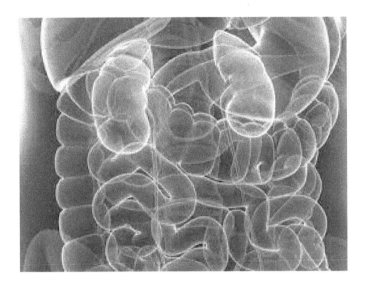

Your doctor can test the function of your kidney with:

- Routine blood examination
- Blood pressure inspections
- Medicines

As the kidneys have such a vital function, people with kidney disease require care. Kidney failure's key treatments are:

Dialysis: This treatment assists the body to clean the blood (doing the function which the kidneys are no longer able to do).

A computer constantly filters the blood for you during hemodialysis. People also undergo this medication for kidney disease 3 to 4 days a week at a hospital or dialysis center. Using a catheter and dialysis fluid, peritoneal dialysis filters the blood in a somewhat different manner. People will do their care at home, often.

Kidney transplantation: Doctors insert a new kidney in your body to take on the function of your weakened organs during kidney transplantation surgery. A dead donor or a live donor may be an acquaintance or family member, maybe the source of this good kidney. With one good kidney, individuals can survive well.

Slowing down of CKD

Chronic kidney disease (CKD) has no remedy, but medication will reduce the negative effects and keep them from becoming worse.

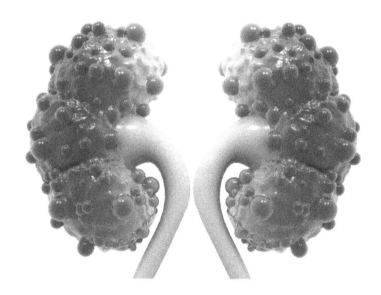

Your condition would rely on your CKD stage.

The primary treatments are:

- To support you remain as safe as possible, lifestyle improvements.
- Medicine to manage related conditions, such as high cholesterol and blood pressure.
- Dialysis-treatment to mimic some of the functions of the kidney that may be needed in advanced CKD (stage 5).
- Kidney transplantation, which may also be expected in advanced CKD (stage 5)
- Modifications of Lifestyle

For patients with kidney failure, the following lifestyle steps are generally recommended:

- No smoking.
- Consuming a balanced, healthy diet
- Limit your salt consumption to less than 6 g a day, which is around 1 tsp.
- Do a routine workout at least 3 hours a week.
- Control of alcohol usage.
- Losing weight if you are obese or overweight
- Stop non-Prescription anti-inflammatory non-steroidal medications (NSAIDs), such as ibuprofen, unless recommended by a medical practitioner. If you have renal failure, these medications may damage the kidneys.

Medicine

Specifically, for CKD, there is no medicine, but medicine may help manage many of the conditions that cause the disease and the problems that may arise as a consequence of it.

To cure or avoid the multiple complications induced by CKD, you need to take medication.

Blood Pressure High

To support the kidneys, proper blood pressure management is important.

People with kidney failure should typically try to keep their blood pressure below 140/90mmHg, but if you already have diabetes, you should manage to get it below 130/80mmHg.

Many forms of blood pressure drugs are essential, but drugs called inhibitors of the angiotensin conversion enzyme (ACE) are also used. For instance, enalapril, ramipril, and lisinopril are used.

ACE inhibitor side effects can include:

- Continuous dry cough
- Dizziness
- Weakness or fatigue

- Headaches

If the negative effects of ACE inhibitors are particularly difficult, a drug called an ARB can be offered instead.

Cholesterol High

A greater likelihood of cardiovascular disease, like heart failure and strokes, are found in individuals with CKD.

This is since some of the factors of kidney illness, including high cholesterol and blood pressure, are the same as those with cardiovascular disease.

To decrease the chance of contracting a cardiovascular disease, medications called statins can be used. Simvastatin and Atorvastatin are examples.

Statin side effects can include:

- Feeling ill
- Headaches
- Diarrhea or constipation
- The pain of muscles and joints
- Retention of Water

If you have kidney failure, you can get swelling of your knees, feet, and hands.

This is because the kidneys do not drain fluid from the blood as easily, allowing it to develop in your tissues (oedema). To further minimize swelling, you might be recommended to limit the normal salt and fluid consumption, including fluids in items such as yogurts and soups.

Diuretics (tablets to make you urinate more) can also be given in certain situations. Dehydration and decreased amounts of potassium and sodium in the blood can be the effects of diuretics.

Anemia

Anemia, a shortage of red blood cells, is acquired by certain individuals with advanced CKD.

Anemia symptoms include:

- Fatigue
- Energy deficit
- Respiratory shortness of air
- Irregular heartbeat (palpitations)

You can be offered doses with a drug named erythropoietin if you have anemia. This is a chemical that generates more red blood cells in the body. If you are still suffering from iron deficiency, iron supplementation can also be prescribed.

Bone problems

You will build-up phosphate in the body if your kidneys are badly compromised; your kidneys will not get rid of it.

Phosphate is essential, along with calcium, for preserving healthy bones. But if the amount of phosphate increases too high, it may disrupt the body's calcium balance and contribute to bone thinning.

You might be recommended to reduce the amount of phosphate-rich food you consume, such as dairy goods, red meat, eggs, and seafood.

If this does not lower the phosphate level sufficiently, drugs called phosphate binders will be offered to you.

There are also low vitamin D levels in certain people with CKD, which is essential for strong bones. You can be offered a supplement named ergocalciferol or cholecalciferol to improve the vitamin D intake if you are poor in vitamin D.

Glomerulonephritis

Swelling of filters within the kidneys, classified as glomerulonephritis, can cause kidney disease.

In certain situations, this happens due to a misguided assault on the kidneys by the immune system.

If the doctor discovers that this is the source of your kidney complications, medication, such as a steroid or a drug named cyclophosphamide, might be used to suppress the function of the immune system.

The kidneys will finally cease functioning for a limited percentage of persons with CKD. It typically happens gradually, but there may be preparation for the next step of the recovery to be scheduled.

When CKD hits this point, one of the alternatives is dialysis. This is a process from which waste materials and extra fluid are separated from the blood.

There are two major dialysis types:

Hemodialysis includes diverting blood through an external system and filtering it before restoring it to the bloodstream.

Peritoneal dialysis requires injecting dialysis fluid inside your tummy into a room to remove waste materials from the blood while they move into vessels covering the inside of your tummy.

Hemodialysis, either at the hospital or at home, is typically performed about 3 days a week. Typically, peritoneal dialysis is performed many times a day.

If you do not get a kidney transplant, you would typically require continuous dialysis care. If your kidney capacity is severely reduced, speak to your doctor about the benefits and drawbacks of each form of dialysis and what form you would choose.

Kidney transplant

A kidney transplant is an approach to dialysis for patients with significantly reduced kidney capacity.

This is also the most common cure for progressive kidney failure, but it requires extensive surgery to avoid the body rejecting the donor organ and taking drugs (immune-suppressants) for the remainder of your life.

You can survive with one kidney; the donor kidneys can be from people who are alive or recently deceased. But there is an organ crisis; you have to wait for months or even years for a replacement.

As you wait for a donor, you will continue to get dialysis. Survival rates are very high for kidney transplants. After 5 years, approximately 90 percent of transplants still perform, and many operate successfully after 10 years and more.

Supportive Care

You would be given supportive care if you chose not to have transplant or dialysis for kidney failure, or you feel that it is not right for you. It is referred to as conservative/palliative care as well.

The goal is to manage and track the signs of kidney disease. It involves therapeutic, practical and medical care, including discussing with the individual with kidney disease and their loved ones on what you feel and how to plan for their death.

The majority of individuals choose supportive care because:

- It isn't easy to benefit or have a decent standard of life from normal treatment.
- May not want to endure the stress of treatment involving dialysis.
- If they have other health problems, the adverse consequences of treatment overshadow the possible benefits.
- They were getting dialysis but preferred the medication to be stopped.
- Dialysis is treated, but their life may be shortened by another serious condition, such as critical heart problems or stroke.
- Supportive care for the kidney would also enable you for a while to experience a respectable life of quality.

Doctors will ensure that you will receive:

- Medicines that maintain the kidney's residual role for as much time as possible
- Medicine for anemia, appetite loss, breathlessness, and itchiness which are some symptoms of renal disease.
- Helping to plan the family and economic issues
- Bereavement aid for their families

What should I do to maintain my kidney's health?

By avoiding or treating health problems that trigger kidney harm, such as heart disease and diabetes, you may protect the kidneys. The actions described below can help to keep your entire body, including your kidneys, safe.

You would want to question your health care professional about your kidneys' health at your next doctor's appointment. There might not be any signs of early kidney failure, but being screened might be the best way to ensure the kidneys are well. Your provider of health services will help determine how much you should be checked.

If you have a UTI, urinary tract infection, which, if left unchecked, will trigger kidney damage, see a specialist right away.

Making good decisions about food

Choose nutritious meals for your body: organic herbs, vegetables, whole-grain foods, and dairy items that are low in fat. Eat things that are nutritious and reduce down sodium and sugar. Per day, strive for less than 2,300 mg. of sodium. Aim to get less than 10% of your total calories from added sugar. Here is a list to help you:

- Pick foods for the body that are balanced.
- Cook with a combination of spices and herbs rather than salt.
- For pizza, choose vegetable toppings like broccoli, spinach, and peppers.
- Rather than frying, consider broiling or baking beef, chicken, and seafood.
- Serve gravy-free items without added fats.
- Try picking items with minimal to no sugar included.
- Try changing from whole milk to two-percent milk.
- Eat whole-grain foods, including whole wheat, oats, brown rice, and maize, every day. For sandwiches and toast, use whole-grain bread; swap white rice with brown rice.
- Interpret labeling on foods. Choose diets poor in saturated fats, salt (sodium), trans fats, added sugar, and cholesterol.
- When eating, slow down. It takes longer than consuming a piece of cake to consume a bowl of popcorn. Instead of having orange juice, eat an orange.

- For a week, consider maintaining a written account about what you are consuming. When you choose to overeat or consume things rich in fat or calories, it will make you see.

- You will want to consult with a dietitian if you have diabetes, elevated blood pressure, or a heart condition to develop a meal plan that fits your needs.

Making regular fitness part of the routine

Exercise on certain days for half an hour or more. Ask the health care professional regarding the forms and quantities of physical exercise right for you if you are not currently involved.

Target a healthy body weight

If you are obese, collaborate to develop a practical weight reduction strategy through your primary care practitioner or dietitian.

Get adequate sleep

Per night, strive for 7 or 8 hours of sleep. If you have difficulty sleeping, take measures to strengthen your sleeping habits.

Stop smoking

If you smoke cigarettes or use other tobacco or nicotine products, please stop. Ask for assistance; you do not have to be alone.

Limit consumption of alcohol

It will raise the blood pressure to consume too much alcohol and consume more calories, contributing to weight gain. Do not drink more than one drink a day if you have to. One beverage is:

- 12 beer ounces

- Five ounces of wine

- Liquor, 1.5 ounce

Try stress-relieving activities

Physical and emotional wellbeing can be enhanced by studying how to handle tension, be calm, and deal with issues. As with mind and body activities such as meditation, yoga, or tai chi, physical exercise can relieve tension.

Control diabetes, heart disease, and blood pressure

The easiest way to defend your kidneys from harm, whether you have diabetes, elevated blood pressure, or heart disease, is to hold blood glucose levels near to the target. An effective approach to treat your diabetes is to control your blood sugar amount.

Hold the figures for blood pressure near to the target. For most persons with diabetes, the blood pressure target is less than 140/90 mm Hg.

Taking all of the medications as indicated. Speak to your health care professional regarding some blood pressure drugs that may protect your kidneys.

Be vigilant of the daily usage of medications for pain. Your kidneys may be impaired by daily usage of anti-inflammatory nonsteroidal drugs, such as ibuprofen.

Hold the cholesterol levels in the goal range to better avoid heart disease and stroke. Your blood produces two types of cholesterol: HDL and LDL. LDL or "poor" cholesterol, which may induce a heart attack, may build up and clog the blood arteries. The "poor" cholesterol in your vessels is eliminated by HDL or "healthy" cholesterol. Another type of fat, called triglycerides, can be measured by a cholesterol test.

Chapter 3- Dialysis and Problems

Working while in dialysis

Work should be enjoyable, help sustain a family, have health care and other rewards, and be socially fulfilling. But, when you hear that you have kidney failure or need to begin dialysis, how can you hold your job? Here are a few suggestions about how your job can be continued.

Understanding what you can do while you have kidney failure at work.

Recognizing what you can and can't do at your workplace is the first move to continuing functioning, whether you operate in offices, a factory, a department store, a store, or outside. Individuals with kidney disease can feel exhaustion or weakness, and the type of work they do may be noticed. You may want to chat about what you should do with your boss or supervisor. For your role, is there something that needs to be changed? Are there various departments that could be more accessible for you? Should you work fewer hours, or work on certain days, perhaps?

They would provide access that has to be safeguarded for persons on dialysis. Vascular access that goes either to the lower or upper arm or upper leg would be essential for anyone who performs hemodialysis procedures, whether in the center or at home. When your work requires physical criteria, ensure your access area is not harmed by this. There is an abdominal catheter of people on peritoneal dialysis that can often be considered while performing hard labor, such as heavy lifting. Your doctor will give you instructions for peritoneal dialysis, like how much weight you can carry.

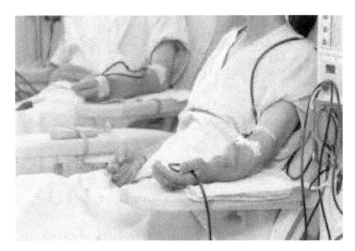

You would still have to make sure to see the doctor arrange appointments for dialysis. If it's an alternative, you may be able to work several days from home.

When you started dialysis, take a temporary leave.

For some purposes, the Department of Labor, Family and Medical Leave Act (FMLA) requires qualified workers to provide qualifying staff with 12 weeks of accrued time off within 12 months. It could be necessary for people with chronic kidney disorder to take advantage of FMLA to get days off to retain their work. When you get a home dialysis access procedure or train, FMLA can aid.

If you need to tend to your medical conditions, you may even start using compensated time off or holiday time. You and your boss should negotiate a voluntary leave of absence, too.

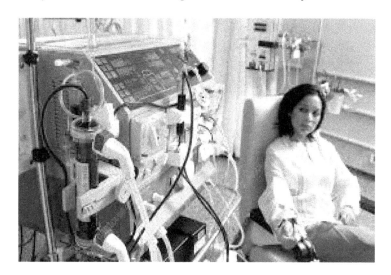

Dialysis options and your job duties

You can have certain choices that could be more conducive to your work and lifestyle than others while heading through dialysis treatments. If you live, where you function, and what sort of career you have will be considerations in determining the option of dialysis therapy. Home dialysis may be the most flexible therapy for dialysis since it is carried out around the work schedule at home.

In center hemodialysis it could be perfect for you if you have a job with flexible working hours, a position that requires you to operate from home, or you operate a night shift.

Nocturnal in-center hemodialysis-This enables you to dialysis overnight at the dialysis center for those who have full-time jobs during the day.

Peritoneal dialysis PD is sometimes administered overnight when you are asleep using an automatic peritoneal dialysis (APD) unit or cycler. This encourages you to be open to work and engage in various events throughout the day. If required, in addition to conducting exchanges at home, peritoneal dialysis patients may also undertake dialysis exchanges in a sterile environment at work throughout the day.

Home hemodialysis (HHD)-Another versatile home dialysis therapy is home hemodialysis since it is carried out in the privacy of your home. The home hemodialysis unit is even smaller than the center system, and treatments can be done at any point of the day or night. Like the PD cycler, the home hemodialysis unit is compact so that you can use it while you are commuting for your work.

Managing tiredness and anemia while you are operating

You might have anemia if you have been fatigued or worn down. Anemia typically occurs in patients with early phases of kidney failure, getting greater as kidney function reduces. Anemia impacts nearly all with end-stage renal disease (ESRD).

Ask the doctor to examine you for anemia if you have experienced symptoms. Your doctor can recommend a medication called erythropoiesis-stimulating agents (ESAs), which act to shape and generate red blood cells if anemia is what you have. EPOGEN ® and Procrit ®, among others, are the terms that can be recommended. When anemia is controlled, you would generally feel fine and will also be able to function.

Returning to work with CKD.

If you'd like to maintain your job if you have kidney problems, you will probably be able to do it. It will sometimes make you feel good, prosperous, and willing to save yourself and family and friends while continuing to function. Educate yourself on which care could be the most work-friendly if you need dialysis. When it comes to manual labor and time-oriented pressures at work, talk with the supervisor about what you are working through and be rational. For even further replies to your questions, chat with an insurance expert.

Chapter 4- Diet

What to consume, what to quit?

How is an eating system essential? Your well-being is influenced by what you consume and drink. It will help regulate your blood pressure and keep at a healthier weight by consuming a nutritious diet minimal in fat and salt.

You will better regulate your blood pressure if you have diabetes by consciously deciding what you consume and drink. It can help keep kidney condition from getting severe by managing hypertension and diabetes.

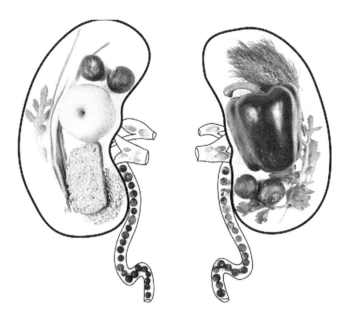

A renal-friendly diet can also help shield your kidneys from more harm. A renal-friendly diet restricts some foods to keep minerals from piling up in the body.

Basics of Balanced Diets

For all meal plans, even a kidney-friendly plan, you need to watch the sum of certain nutrient you eat in, such as:

- Calories
- Protein
- Fat
- Carbohydrate

To ensure you are consuming the correct proportions of these foods, you should drink and eat the appropriate portion sizes. On the "Nutrition Facts" tab are all the details you need to maintain your consumption.

To read all about what is in the stuff you consume, use the nutrition information category on food labels. Food facts inform you how much sugars, fats, proteins, sodium, and minerals are in a portion of food. This will assist you in selecting foods that are heavy in the nutrients required and lower in the nutrients that should be restricted.

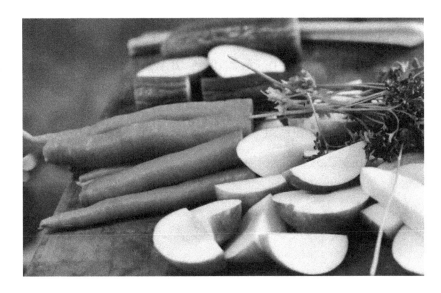

View the nutritional facts; there are some key areas that will give you the information you need:

Calories

The body obtains strength from the calories that you consume and eat.

The calories come from carbohydrates, proteins, and fat. The calories you need can be estimated based on your body size, age, gender, and amount of exercise.

You would also need to adjust how much calories you eat, depending on your weight objectives. The calories eaten will have to be limited to certain persons. Those who need to get more calories might be there. A nutritionist or doctor can help you figure out how many calories are required. To ensure you have the right amount of calories and keep in touch with them, consult with your nutritionist, and establish a meal plan.

Protein

This is one of the principal building blocks of the body. Your body needs protein to grow, regenerate, and keep healthy. It would make the hair, skin, and nails fragile from having very little protein. But consuming excess protein can be a problem as well. In order to keep healthy to help you feel the strongest, you'll need to adjust the amount of protein you eat.

The amount of protein you require may be determined based on body size, exercise level, or health conditions. Many clinicians prescribe that people with kidney problems reduce protein intake or change their sources of protein. This is because it would be hard for the kidneys to work because of a very high protein diet, creating more damage.

Consult the dietitian regarding the amount of protein you can consume and which types of protein are best for you. Remember that it is not possible to eat limitless amounts only because a diet is poor in proteins.

Low protein-level foods:

- Pasta
- Vegetables
- Fruits
- Bread

Foods with a higher protein content:

- Red meat
- Poultry
- Eggs
- Fish

The following are important to monitor and to encourage a kidney diet:

Sodium

Sodium is found in many foods. The plurality of individuals think of sodium and salt as synonymous. Salt, though, is, in reality, a chloride and sodium compound. The food we consume may include salt or may include other sources of sodium. Due to additional salt, refined foods also have higher sodium levels.

It is one of the three main electrolytes (the other two being chloride and potassium) in the body. The fluids moving inside and outside of the cells and tissues of the body are regulated by electrolytes. Sodium provides a contribution to:

- Blood volume and Blood pressure control
- Regulating nerve activity and contraction of muscles
- Regulating acid-base blood balance
- Balancing the amount of fluid contained or eliminated by the body

Why should sodium consumption be controlled by kidney patients?

For patients with renal failure, too much salt may be dangerous since their kidneys cannot remove extra salt from the body properly. As they concentrate sodium and fluid in the bloodstream and tissues, this may induce:

- Excessive thirst
- Edema: a swelling of the hands, legs, and face
- Blood pressure is high
- Heart failure: The heart will overwork with extra fluid in the blood, rendering it swollen and sluggish.
- Breathlessness: fluid in the lungs will build up, making it hard to breathe.

How can patients be expected to control their consumption of sodium?

- Always read the food labels. They list the sodium content.
- Pay careful attention to sizes for serving.
- Use fresh, instead of packaged meat products.
- Pick fresh vegetables and fruits.

- Stop refined goods.
- Compare companies and choose the lowest-sodium products.
- Using spices that do not mention in their title 'salt' (garlic powder rather than garlic salt.)
- Make homemade food and avoid salt.
- Limit the average amount of sodium to 400 milligrams per every meal and 150 milligrams per every snack.

Potassium

Potassium and the role it plays:

Potassium is present in all of the things that we consume and is naturally found in the body as well. In holding the pulse normal and the muscles functioning properly, potassium plays a part. For the preservation of electrolyte and fluid equilibrium in the blood, potassium is also required. The kidneys aid in keeping the body's proper level of potassium and remove unnecessary levels.

Why do patients with kidney disease control their intake of potassium?

They will no longer expel surplus potassium as the kidneys malfunction, so potassium builds up inside the body of the patient. High blood potassium is recognized as hyperkalemia, which may trigger:

- Muscular fatigue
- An abnormal heart rhythm
- Weak pulse
- Heart attacks

How can people control their consumption of potassium?

A patient must control the volume of potassium that reaches the body as the kidneys in his body no longer balance potassium.

Here are some tips:

Talk regarding developing a meal schedule with a dietitian.

- Restrict foods rich in potassium.

Consume no more than 8 ounces a day of milk along with dairy goods.

Pick fresh vegetables and fruits.

Stop salt substitutes and potassium seasonings.

Read labels and restrict potassium chloride in processed goods.

Look at the serving size.

Keep a diet log.

Phosphorus

Phosphorus and the role it plays:

Phosphorus is important in the preservation and growth of bones. Phosphorus frequently helps grow connective tissues along with organs and aids in the movement of muscles. As phosphorus-containing food is eaten and digested, phosphorus is absorbed by the small intestine to be contained in the bones.

Why should phosphorus consumption be controlled by kidney patients?

Normal functioning kidneys can extract excess phosphorus from the blood. The kidneys cannot expel surplus phosphorus if kidney activity is compromised. A high concentration of phosphorus can pull calcium from your bones and make them fragile. This often results in harmful calcium concentrations in the lungs, skin, blood vessels, and heart.

How can patients be expected to control their consumption of phosphorus?

Phosphorus is found in most foods. Therefore, to better control phosphorus amounts, patients with impaired kidney function may consult with a renal dietician.

Tips for helping to retain phosphorus at healthy levels:

- Know which foods have less phosphorus.
- Pay careful attention to the size of servings.
- Eat smaller amounts of food that are rich in protein.

- Eat vegetables and fruits.
- Enquire your doctor regarding using phosphate binders during meals.
- Stop processed goods with added phosphorus. In labels, check for phosphorus or terms with "PHOS".
- Keep a diet log

Fluids

For people in the later phases of CKD Chronic Kidney Disease, fluid management is important since regular fluid intake can contribute to fluid build-up inside the body that may become harmful. People on dialysis also have reduced flow of urine, so additional fluid in the body will place undue pressure on the lungs and heart of the person.

The fluid allocation of a patient, based on urinary production and dialysis conditions, is measured on an individual basis. Pursuing the fluid intake requirements set by your nutritionist is important.

To monitor the consumption of fluids:

- Don't consume more alcohol than what is recommended by your doctors
- List all food items that melt at normal temperature (popsicles, jelly, etc.)
- Be aware of the quantity of liquids used during cooking

Chapter 5- Frequently Asked Questions

Does dialysis trigger weight loss for me?

The machine may indicate you are shedding weight when you begin dialysis. The weight loss, though, maybe induced by the fluid loss that is taken out by dialysis. Over time, fluid might have accumulated up that the kidneys could not adequately perform this task. When you undergo dialysis, you can even lose a small amount of weight, and the build-up of contaminants in your bloodstream (before beginning dialysis, the kidneys do not function well) will decrease the appetite. So, you may find that you aren't eating normally when you initiate dialysis for the first time. It may require a couple of weeks of continuous dialysis (to eliminate from your blood all the "added up" or unwanted toxins) before you begin to feel healthier, and your appetite increases or goes back to normal.

May I eat from restaurants?

Alright, but note the limits of your food and liquids. When cooking the meals, most restaurants incorporate the salt. Try to refrain from applying salt to the meal. Ask the dietitian while dining out for advice about proper diet choices.

Can I drink sodas and other beverages?

Any pop/soda forms may be rich in phosphorus content. All colas (both regular and diet) include phosphorus and must be restricted and prevented. Dr. Pepper's and a few other carbonated ice teas also incorporate phosphorus and, therefore, should be handled just like cola. There is very little to no phosphorus in citrus and similar flavored sodas, and they are good to drink (i.e., lemon-lime, root beer, cherry, peach, etc.). Restrict the regular quantity of wine and alcoholic beverages to not more than a single small bottle. Alcohol includes phosphorus, which, like cola, should be restricted (1 may be suggested per day). Owing to their additional vitamins, nutrients, and spices, which dialysis cannot kill and can build up in the bloodstream, all energy beverages (i.e., Red bull) or athletic beverages (i.e., Gatorade) should be prohibited at all times.

May I take my mineral, vitamin, and herbal supplements?

Your doctor or nutritionist will recommend a particular multi-vitamin for persons on dialysis to use every day before you begin dialysis. Unless indicated by the dietitian, no other nutrient, herbal, and mineral supplementation should be taken. Please let them know right away whether you are already taking any supplements not recommended by the nephrologist or dietitian.

I'm a vegetarian. If I start dialysis, will I be okay?

You can adopt a vegetarian diet during dialysis, although it may require some more effort to ensure you consume adequate protein. Many forms of vegetable protein are often very rich in phosphorus and potassium, which must be restricted for dialysis for most citizens. The strongest protein sources come from beef and other items of animal origin. The vegetarians of Lacto-ova can consume sufficient protein from eggs and dairy products. Without an inadequate consumption of potassium or phosphorus, vegetarians will find it very challenging to eat a suitable protein volume from vegetarian sources.

I'm diabetic. When on dialysis, will my blood sugar be hard to control?

The majority of people with diabetes who have initiated dialysis have now noticed that their sugar is simpler to regulate now. This doesn't indicate that after beginning dialysis, it would be okay for people with diabetes to raise their sugar consumption and to avoid taking oral/insulin diabetic tablets. To avoid any problems due to inadequate blood sugar regulation, it is also really necessary to control the blood sugar level while on dialysis. You will need to track the blood sugar by selecting peritoneal dialysis, mostly because of the dextrose which is injected into the solution for peritoneal dialysis.

Why is there a weird taste on my tongue?

Many contaminants will build up inside your blood until dialysis is prescribed by your nephrologist, so your kidneys no longer function properly. This toxin build-up will trigger you to get a metallic flavor inside your mouth. Typically, this may go away after you undergo dialysis, but if you continually skip appointments or cut the recommended medication period, it will return.

Why does my hair fall out?

Hair is made mainly of protein. Any kidney specialists think that it is triggered by protein deficiency. Your body will continue to inject protein in your urine as you begin to experience kidney failure, producing less protein in your blood. Besides, it is advised that certain persons who are not yet on dialysis continue to reduce their protein consumption to place less burden on their residual activity of the kidney. This could be the beginning of hair loss. They tend to consume much protein until people undergo dialysis. Dialysis itself may eliminate any protein from the blood. Other experts suggest that loss of hair in patients on dialysis may be related to stress.

Why do I have a loss of appetite?

When the kidneys struggle to clean waste out of the blood, lack of appetite is common. To remain safe and avoid muscle loss, it is vital to get adequate protein and calories.

If you have a poor appetite:

- Eat small, quick meals and calorie-dense snacks (every 2 to 3 hours) during your day.
- Eat your largest meal when your hunger is great. If you're not starving at night, have your full meal at lunch or breakfast.
- If you are away from home for the day, at counseling, meetings, or college, take treats with you. Options include crackers and cheese, a mini muffin, or one half of a sandwich.
- Schedule meals and snacks-if you do not feel hungry set an alarm as a prompt to feed.
- Experiment with new recipes, such as trying frozen foods instead of a hot lunch, for example.
- Create a list of recipes that are simple or favorite and look at it when you are not sure what to consume.
- Try to take a stroll to get some fresh air, which might make you feel hungry.
- Contact your dietitian regarding seeking a liquid supplement that is kidney safe.

Let every bite count. Add additional calories and protein:

- Add margarine to rice, pasta, crackers, vegetables, and toast.
- Using toast, bread, and crackers with butter, jelly, margarine, or cream cheese.
- In soups, pasta or potatoes, mix cooked, chicken ground beef, or turkey.
- For fruits, salads, or casseroles, incorporate the cheese.
- Add eggs or tuna to salad.

- On crackers, toast or fruit, add peanut butter.
- For soups, stews, or stir-fry, incorporate tofu.
- Eat cottage cheese, which is unsalted with fruit.
- Regularly use "good" fats. Attempt dipping toast in olive oil.
- Sauté meals in olive oil or canola.
- For salads and vegetables, apply low-salt dressings.
- Drink calorie-containing beverages.
- On desserts and fruits, use whipped topping.

Changing Diet?

A reference for persons at an early stage of kidney failure.

It is necessary for anyone to enjoy a balanced diet. For those with kidney disease, it is extremely crucial. Your diet will help delay the development of your kidney disease. What you consume plays an important role in:

- Keeping/attaining a good weight
- Maintaining lower blood pressure
- Managing the rate of blood glucose when you have diabetes
- Managing amounts of cholesterol
- It is critical for people in the early stages of kidney disease to adopt a healthy diet and lifestyle. Helpful hints are described below for following a healthy diet:
- Eat periodic meals
- Eating a range of foods from all of the food classes
- Stop applying salt and serving high-salt foods

Is exercise meaningful?

Daily activity is important. This improves with:

- Regulation of blood pressure
- The management of a good weight
- Treatment of diabetes
- Power and health

It is advised that people workout several days of the week for 30 minutes. If you cannot work out consistently for 30 minutes, then many shorter sessions a day is often helpful. Healthy fitness means walking at a speed that is easy for you to speak at. This, this, Grass mowing, dance, medium speed swimming, or cycling may be included. Before initiating a special workout, contact a doctor.

Breakfasts

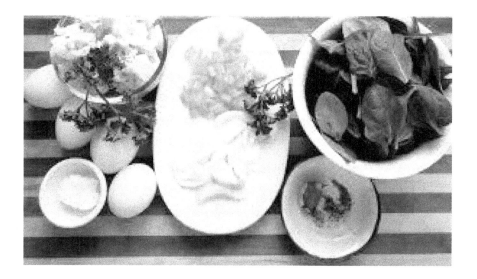

1. Herbed Omelet

Makes: 2 portions

Serving size is ½ omelet

Ingredients

- Vegetable oil, 1 ½ tsp
- Chopped onion, 1 tbsp.
- Eggs, 4
- Water, 2 tbsp.
- Basil, ¼ tsp
- Tarragon, ⅛ tsp
- Parsley, ¼ tsp (optional)

Directions

1. Beat all eggs and add spices. And the water in it.
2. In an 8" frying pan, heat oil on medium heat, add in onions and fry. Remove fried onio0n from pan.
3. Pour beaten egg mixture into a heated frying pan on medium heat.

4. When the omelet sets, lift with a flat spoon to let the uncooked egg mixture flow to the bottom of the pan.
5. When the omelet sets completely, top the omelet with the sautéed onion and move to a serving dish.

Nutritional Analysis

195 Calories | 14 gr Protein | 15 gr total Fat | 0 gr Carbohydrate

157 mg Sodium | 157 mg Potassium | 214 mg Phosphorus

2. Fruit Omelet

Makes: 4 portions

Serving size is ¼ omelet

Ingredients

- Frozen strawberries, 2 cups, thawed
- Sugar, 1 tbsp. (optional)
- Eggs, 4, separated
- Lemon juice, 1 tbsp.
- Unsalted butter, 1 tbsp. (or margarine)

Directions

1. Heat oven to 375°f.

2. Put strawberries in a bowl and sprinkle with sugar; let them stand.

3. In a medium bowl beat egg whites until stiff.

4. In a separate bowl, beat the yolks and juice of a lemon. Fold the stiff egg whites into beaten yolks till no yellow streaks show.

5. In an oven-safe skillet (10"), melt butter. Into the skillet, pour the egg mixture, coat sides by tilting pan. For 5 minutes, cook on low heat.

6. When the mixture is set on the pan's bottom, bake in the oven for 5 more minutes.

7. Onto a heated plate, place omelet. Spread strawberries on the hot omelet. Cut into wedges and Serve hot.

Nutritional Analysis

198 Calories | 8 gr Protein | 9 gr total Fat | 24 gr Carbohydrate

125 mg Sodium | 430 mg Potassium | 141 mg Phosphorus.

3. Old Fashioned Pancakes

Makes: 4 small pancakes

Serving size is 1 pancake

Ingredients

- All-purpose flour, ½ cup
- Egg, 1, beaten
- Granulated sugar, ¼ cup
- Baking powder, ¼ tsp
- 2% milk, ¼ cup, plus ¼ cup water
- Vegetable oil, 1 tbsp.

Directions

1. In a bowl, mix the first four ingredients. Mix thoroughly. Add in milk. Add water for thinner batter for pancakes or less for thicker pancakes.
2. In a skillet, heat oil. Pour batter on the skillet ¼ cup at a time.
3. Cook each side until brown.

Nutritional Analysis

165 Calories | 4 gr Protein | 5 gr total Fat | 26 gr Carbohydrates

58 mg Sodium | 57 mg Potassium | 64 mg Phosphorus

4. French Toast

Makes: 4 portions

Serving size is 1 slice

Ingredients

- Egg whites, 4 large, slightly beaten
- 1% milk, ¼ cup
- Cinnamon, ½ tsp
- Allspice, ¼ tsp
- White bread, 4 slices (maybe toasted)
- Margarine, 1 tbsp.

Directions

1. To egg whites, Add milk, allspice, and cinnamon.

2. One slice at a time Dip bread into the batter.

3. In a heated skillet, melt margarine Place a slice of bread on the skillet.

4. Fry bread on both sides till golden brown.

5. Drizzle with syrup and serve hot (sugar-free if diabetic).

Nutritional Analysis

125 Calories | 7 gr Protein | 5 gr total Fat | 14 gr Carbohydrate

194 mg Sodium | 128 mg Potassium | 61 mg Phosphorus

5. Corn Pudding

Makes: 6 portions

Serving size is ½ cup

Ingredients

- Kernel corn, 2 cups fresh cut or canned
- Eggs, 3 slightly beaten or egg substitute, ¾ cup
- 1% milk, ½ cup
- Onion, ⅓ cup, finely chopped
- Water, ½ cup
- Butter, 1 tbsp., melted
- Granulated sugar, 1 tsp
- Black pepper or white, 1 tsp

Directions

1. Heat oven to 350°f.
2. Mix all ingredients in a bowl.
3. Take a 1 ½-quart casserole dish, grease it and Pour the mixture in it.
4. Place the casserole dish in a low pan filled with 1 inch of hot water.
5. Bake until center sets or a knife inserted in comes out clean or for about 40-45 minutes.
6. Let it stand at room temperature for 10 minutes before serving.

Nutritional Analysis

120 Calories | 6 gr Protein | 5 gr total Fat | 17 gr Carbohydrate

61 mg Sodium | 234 mg Potassium | 122 mg Phosphorus

6. Kale and Cheddar Frittata

Makes: 4 portions

Serving size is 1 wedge

Ingredients

- Large eggs, 8

- Olive oil, 2 tbsp.
- Lacinato kale, 4 oz. (about ½ bunch), tough stems removed and cut into ribbons
- Kosher salt, ¼ tsp
- Ground black pepper, ¼ tsp
- Red pepper flakes, ¼ tsp crushed
- Garlic, 2 cloves, minced
- English cheddar, 1 oz, shredded (or any sharp cheese)

Directions

1. Heat oven to 350°F.
2. Beat the eggs in a small bowl and put aside.
3. In an oven-safe skillet, heat the oil on medium heat. Add the kale, black pepper, salt, and red pepper and heat, occasionally stirring, until the kale starts to droop. Include the garlic and simmer for 2 more minutes. Take away from the heat.
4. Transfer the beaten eggs into the hot skillet and give it a quick mix with the kale. Scatter the cheese on top and roast in the oven till the eggs are set, for about 10 minutes. Portion into 4 equal wedges and serve.

Nutritional Analysis

248 Calories | 20 gr Fat | 4 gr Carbohydrates | 16 gr Protein

252 mg Sodium | 233 mg Phosphorus | 281 mg Potassium

7. Spanish Tortilla or Omelet

Makes: 8 portions

Serving size is ⅛ tortilla

Ingredients

- Potatoes, golden, 5, small

- Olive oil, 1 cup, (½ cup will be left and reused)
- Onion, 1 large, halved, and sliced
- Red bell pepper, 1 small, diced
- Black pepper, ¼ tsp, ground
- Eggs, 8, medium
- Salt, ¼ tsp

Directions

1. Preheat oven to 400°F.
2. Split the potatoes halfway across. Put the flat surface of each half of it on the chopping board and cut it thinly.
3. Top the potatoes in a small saucepan with water. Cook the potato slices until they are partly tender, around 5 minutes.
4. Drain the potatoes and pat carefully before frying.
5. Heat olive oil over low heat in a low nonstick skillet that is ovenproof.
6. Include bell pepper and onion and fry for five minutes. Include the potato slices and sauté until the potatoes are lightly browned around 7-8 minutes.
7. Sprinkle with black pepper over the vegetables and swirl to combine. Drain the extra cooking oil from the pan and transfer it into a container. Cooldown the vegetables marginally.
8. In a big mixing dish, beat the eggs and salt.
9. Shift the strained cooked vegetables into the beaten egg.
10. Transfer 1 tbsp. of the remaining oil to the pan and cook over medium heat.
11. Tilt the pan to coat the pan's whole bottom (helps stop the eggs from sticking).
12. Place the mixture of vegetables and eggs into the heated skillet. Mix with the spoon and allow the egg to thicken a little bit for 3-5 minutes.
13. Lower the heat and finish cooking the omelet for another 10 minutes. At the same time, be

using a spatula to check that the edges of the omelet do not cling to the skillet. Shake the skillet softly with its handle a minute or two to ensure that the omelet is loose and the bottom does not stick.

14. Move the skillet to the oven while the top is also a little undercooked, yet you can tell the bottom is strong. Bake until the top is cooked for 7-8 minutes.

15. Remove from the oven and put on a flat plate.

16. Cover the top and turn it over with another flat plate, exposing a golden-brown surface.

17. Serve instantly with a salad or set aside for later meals

Nutritional Analysis

265 Calories | 18 gr Fat | 18 gr Carbohydrate | 7 gr Protein

166 mg Sodium | 114 mg Phosphorus | 355 mg Potassium

8. Egg Salad on Homemade Biscuit

Makes: 4 portions

Serving size is ¼ egg salad + 1 biscuit

Ingredients

For Mayonnaise: (makes 1 cup, can be stored for up to 10 days)

- Medium egg, 1
- Lemon juice, 2 tsp, freshly squeezed
- Sunflower, 1 cup (or other vegetable oil)
- For biscuit: (makes 6)
- All-purpose flour, 1 cup
- Baking powder, 1 ½ tsp
- Sugar, 1 tbsp.
- Cold butter, ¼ cup (chilled in the freezer for 20 min)

- Whole milk, ⅓ cup
- Large egg, 1

For Egg Salad:

- Medium eggs, 4
- Carrots, ¼ cup, grated
- Celery, ¾ cup, diced
- Red onion, ¼ cup
- Cornichon pickles, 4
- Homemade mayonnaise, ¼ cup
- Dijon mustard, 1 tsp
- Fresh dill, 1 tbsp., chopped
- Black pepper, ¼ tsp, freshly ground
- Fresh parsley, 1 tbsp., chopped

Directions

For Mayonnaise:

1. Into the blender, break an egg.
2. If used, include the salt and lemon juice.
3. Pour a constant stream of sunflower oil out of a glass container into the blender at medium level.
4. Raise the speed as the solution thickens.
5. When you steadily finish pouring the oil, keep blending. Put it aside, Set it back.

For Biscuit:

1. Heat the oven to 425 ° F and line with parchment paper, a baking sheet.

2. In a big bowl, mix the flour, sugar, salt, and baking powder. Mix thoroughly. Put aside.

3. Break the butter into little bits. Rub the butter into the flour, using your fingertips or a pastry cutter only until the mixture imitates coarse crumbs.

4. Include the egg and milk. Stir until they're all mixed.

5. Move the biscuit dough to a well-floured table. Lightly knead. If it becomes too sticky, incorporate the flour till it's manageable.

6. Using both hands to stretch the dough till the mixture is an inch thick. Straight down the pastry, push a biscuit cutter, and transfer the Biscuit to the prepared baking tray.

7. Repeat until you've got about 6 biscuits, 1/2 inch away on the baking tray.

8. Bake for around 12 minutes or till the tops are golden brown.

For Egg Salad:

1. In a medium pan, put the eggs and cover them with water (1 inch above the eggs).

2. Bring it to a boil.

3. Turn the heat off, cover the pan, and let it stay for 12 minutes. Then, drain.

4. For 2 minutes, immerse eggs in cold water.

5. Peel the eggs and chop them. Add in a medium bowl.

6. Attach sliced celery, onion, pickles, and carrots.

7. Adding 1/4 cup Dijon mustard, homemade mayo, salt, herbs, and pepper (if using). Mix thoroughly.

8. Serve cut in half on a warm biscuit.

Nutritional Analysis

379 Calories | 28 gr Fat | 22 gr Carbohydrate | 10 gr Protein

274 mg Sodium | 167 mg Phosphorus | 210 mg Potassium

9. Apple and Zucchini Harvest Muffins

Makes: 12 muffins

Serving size is 1 muffin

Ingredients

- Whole wheat pastry flour, 1 cup (or all-purpose flour if unavailable)
- All-purpose flour, ½ cup
- Ground flax seeds, ¼ cup
- Baking powder, one tsp
- Baking soda, ½ tsp
- Ground cinnamon, 1 tsp
- Canola oil, ⅓ cup
- Sugar, ¼ cup
- Apple cider vinegar, 1 tbsp.
- Egg, 1
- Unsweetened applesauce, ½ cup
- Molasses, 1 tbsp.
- Zucchini, grated, 1 medium (about 1 cup)
- Shredded apple, ½ cup

Directions

1. Heat oven to 425°F.

2. Brush a muffin tray with nonstick spray for baking. In a big bowl, mix the flour, cinnamon, baking soda, flax seeds, baking powder together.

3. Whisk the oil, apple cider vinegar, sugar, egg, molasses, and applesauce together in another container until well mixed. Mix in the apples and the zucchini.

4. Put dry ingredients together and add the wet ingredients. Stir to mix a few times. To the prepared muffin cups, add batter.

5. Cook at 425 ° F for 5 minutes and then reduce the oven temperature to 350 ° F.

6. Serve warm.

Nutritional Analysis

178 Calories | 8 gr Fat | 25 gr Carbohydrate | 3 gr Protein

157 mg Sodium | 59 mg Phosphorus | 127 mg Potassium

10. Banana Chocolate Chip Muffins

Makes: 12 muffins

Serving size is 1 muffin

Ingredients

- Over-ripe bananas, 2 large, mashed
- Large egg, 1
- Light brown sugar, ⅓ cup
- Olive oil, ¼ cup
- Plain yogurt, 2 tbsp.
- Vanilla extract, 1 tsp
- All-purpose flour, unbleached, 1 cup
- Sea salt, ¼ tsp
- Baking soda, ½ tsp

- Nutmeg, ¼ tsp
- Almonds, ⅓ cup sliced
- Dark chocolate chips, ⅔ cup

Directions

1. Heat the oven to 350°F.
2. Brush muffin molds with oil or fill with muffin liners.
3. Mix together bananas, egg, oil, and sugar in a medium-sized mixing bowl and stir well.
4. Include vanilla and yogurt and mix with a spatula until smooth.
5. Add in the flour ¼ cup at a time, adding baking soda and salt in between additions.
6. Mix all thoroughly.
7. Sprinkle chocolate chips and almonds.
8. Bake for 12 minutes approximately. Serve and enjoy.

Nutritional Analysis

149 Calories | 7 gr Fat | 19 gr Carbohydrates | 3 gr Protein

110 mg Sodium | 44 mg Phosphorus | 140 mg Potassium

First Course

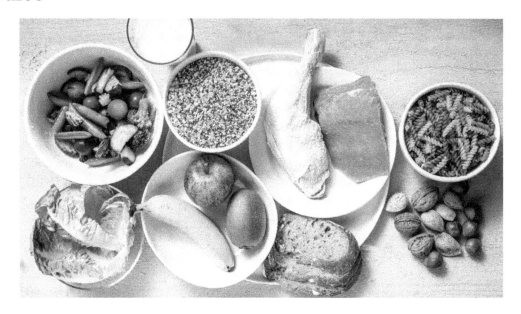

11. Curry Chicken

Makes: 6 portions

Serving size is 3-oz

Ingredients

- Chicken, 1 whole, cut in small parts, skin removed
- Lemon juice, ¼ cup
- Dry thyme, ½ tsp
- Curry powder, 2 tsp
- Onion, 1 medium, chopped
- Garlic clove, 1 medium chopped (optional)
- Black pepper, ½ tsp
- Vegetable, 2 tbsp. (or olive oil)
- Water, 1 cup

Directions

1. Pour lemon juice on cleaned Chicken and wash it.

2. Combine seasoning together in a bowl and rub it on chicken parts.

3. Marinate the seasoned chicken overnight in the refrigerator (can be used after 1 hour).

4. In a saucepan, heat oil, fry seasoned Chicken till browned.

5. From the marinated bowl, Rinse remaining seasoning with water.

6. Pour this remaining marinade over browned Chicken. Let cook on low heat until tender.

7. Place over hot rice and serve.

Nutritional Analysis

323 Calories | 21 gr Protein | 24 gr total Fat | 5 gr Carbohydrate

93 mg Sodium | 317 mg Potassium | 214 mg Phosphorus

12. Spicy Lamb

Makes: 4 portions

Serving size is 3-oz

Ingredients

- 1 lamb leg (trimmed for roasting)
- Vegetable oil, ¼ cup
- Garlic powder, 1 ½ tbsp.
- Dry mustard, 3 tsp

Directions

1. Mix ingredients for the marinade: garlic powder, oil, and mustard.

2. Rub leg of lamb with marinade thoroughly; refrigerate overnight or for 6-8 hours.

3. Heat barbecue spit Adjust meat on it and bake drizzling meat constantly with marinade until 170°F on a meat thermometer or for 30 minutes per pound.

Nutritional Analysis

289 Calories | 24 gr Protein | 6 gr total Fat | 3 gr Carbohydrate

144 mg Sodium | 423 mg Potassium | 237 mg Phosphorus

13. Special Pizza

Makes: 10 slices

Serving size is 1 slice (5 ½" x 3" x ¼")

Ingredients for crust

- Active dry yeast, 1 tsp
- Granulated sugar, 1 tbsp.
- Water, 1 cup
- All-purpose flour, 2 cups
- Vegetable shortening, 2 tbsp.

Directions

1. In a mixing bowl, mix flour, sugar, and yeast.
2. Add in shortening to the above ingredients; mix all together using a fork.
3. Include water in little quantities while mixing together with the fork until the mixture combines well together and follows the fork around the bowl.
4. Allow the dough to rest after covering for about 15 minutes.

Ingredients for Pizza:

- Ground beef, ½ pound lean (or Chicken or turkey)
- Italian seasoning, ½ tsp
- Tomato paste, ¼ cup
- Onion powder, ½ tsp
- Chili powder, 1 tsp

- Garlic powder, ½ tsp
- Italian seasoning, 1 tsp
- Water vegetable oil, ½ cup
- Sharp cheddar cheese, 4 oz. reduced-fat, grated
- Green peppers, ½ cup, diced
- Onions, ½ cup, diced

Directions

1. Heat oven to 425°f.
2. Sauté ground meat in a frying pan. Add onion powder, Italian seasoning, and garlic
3. powder; stir continuously until meat is brown.
4. Drain the oil by Placing meat onto paper towels.
5. In a small bowl, prepare the pizza sauce by blending the tomato paste, Italian seasoning, chili powder, and water. Put aside.
6. Take out the rested dough, grease fingers, and pizza pan. Stretch dough on the pan evenly.
7. Evenly Pour sauce over pizza dough; scatter with ½ cup of cheese.
8. Bake in the heated oven for around 15-20 minutes.
9. Take out from oven; include ground beef, onions, green peppers, and remaining cheese.
10. Put back in the oven for an added 10 minutes. Serve hot.

Nutritional Analysis

196 Calories | 11 gr Protein | 7 gr total Fat | 24 gr Carbohydrate

144 mg Sodium | 188 mg Potassium | 31 mg Phosphorus

14. Slow-Cooked Lemon Chicken

Makes: 4 portions

Serving size is 4 oz.

Ingredients

- Dried oregano, 1 tsp
- Ground black pepper, ¼ tsp
- Butter, unsalted, 2 tbsps.
- Chicken breast, 1 pound, boneless, skinless
- Chicken broth, ¼ cup, low sodium
- Water, ¼ cup
- Lemon juice, 1 tbsp.
- Garlic, minced, 2 cloves
- Fresh basil, 1 tsp, chopped

Directions

1. In a small bowl, mix oregano and grounded black pepper. Coat mixture on the chicken.
2. In a medium skillet, soften the butter over medium heat. Cook the chicken in the melted butter till it is golden brown and then shift the chicken to the slow cooker.
3. To loosen the brown bits stuck in the skillet, pour water, chicken broth, garlic, and lemon juice in the skillet, get it to a boil. Pour this over the browned chicken.
4. Close the slow cooker and set on low for 5 hours or on high for 2½ hours.
5. Baste chicken and Add basil. For an additional 15-30 minutes, Cover and cook on high or until chicken is soft and tender.

Nutritional Analysis

197 Calorie | 26 gr Protein | 9 gr Total Fat | 1 gr Carbohydrates

57 mg Sodium | 251 mg Phosphorus | 412 mg Potassium

15. Classic Beef Stroganoff with Egg Noodles

Makes: 6 portions

Serving size is 10 oz.

Ingredients

- Onions, 1 cup, finely diced
- Egg, beaten, 1
- Worcestershire sauce, 2 tbsp., reduced-sodium
- Breadcrumbs, ¼ cup
- Mayonnaise, 1 tbsp.
- Tomato sauce, 1 tbsp., no salt added
- Ground beef, 1 pound
- Canola oil, 3 tbsp.
- Flour, 2 tbsp.
- Water, 3 cups
- Black pepper, 1 tsp, freshly ground
- Better than bouillon beef, 4 tsp, reduced-sodium
- Sour cream, ¼ cup
- 2 tbsp. chives
- Wide egg noodles, ½ package (12oz package), cooked
- Butter, unsalted, 2 tbsp., cold and cubed
- Parsley, ¼ cup

- Rosemary, chopped, 1 tbsp.

Directions

1. Mix the first six ingredients and half tsp black pepper in a big bowl. Add in the ground beef and mix thoroughly. Make 16 meatballs of the same size.

2. Cook stroganoff meatballs in a big frypan until browned on medium heat. Shift all meatballs to one area and add oil and flour to the same pan and stir until well-combined. Add the remaining black pepper, water, and bouillon, and then keep stirring until sauce thickens, for 10 minutes.

3. Take off the heat and mix in chives and sour cream, then serve over egg noodles.

Pasta:

1. To a large pan, add egg noodles with 2 tbsp. of water, heat and mix until warm, then take off the heat. Mix in butter, rosemary, and parsley until everything is well incorporated.

Nutritional Analysis

490 Calories | 20gr Protein | 32 gr Total Fat | 30 gr Carbohydrates

598 mg Sodium | 230 mg Phosphorus 230 | 423 mg Potassium

16. Roast Pork Loin with Sweet and Tart Apple Stuffing

Makes: 6 portions

Serving size is 2.5–3 oz. or 1/6 loin

Ingredients

Cherry marmalade glaze:

- Dried cherries, ¼ cup

- Orange marmalade, ½ cup sugar-free

- Nutmeg, 1/8 tsp

- Apple juice, ¼ cup

- Cinnamon, 1/8 tsp

Apple stuffing:

- Canola oil, 2 tbsp.

- Hawaiian rolls, 2 cups packed cubed (or any white bread)

- Granny smith, ½ cup, finely diced (honey crisp or macintosh apple)

- Butter, 2 tbsp., unsalted

- Onions, finely diced, 2 tbsp.

- Celery, finely diced, 2 tbsp.

- Fresh thyme, 1 tbsp., (or dried thyme, ½ tsp)

- Black pepper, 1 tsp

- Chicken stock, low-sodium, ½ cup

Roast pork loin:

- Pork loin, 1 pound, boneless

- Butcher twine, two 18-inch pieces

Directions

Glaze Cherry Marmalade:

1. In a small pan, mix all the glaze ingredients on medium-high heat till marmalade is liquefied and starts to bubble. Take off heat and put aside.

2. Heat oven to 400° F.

Apple Stuffing:

3. In a large sauté pan, slightly fry all ingredients in oil on medium-high heat for 2–3 minutes except for chicken stock.

4. Gradually add chicken stock until moist, but not too wet. (may not be needed as it may depend on how much juice is released from the apples during cooking.)

5. Take off from heat and cool it to room temperature.

Pork Loin:

6. In the meantime, form several pockets by cutting five slits along the length of the loin, about 1 inch apart

7. Fill each pocket with around 2 tbsp. of stuffing (saving around a half cup)

8. To keep the stuffing in place, tie the twine around the loin as needed.

9. Put remainder stuffing on a baking tray, top with tied stuffed pork, and bake for 45 minutes at 400° F, check with an internal temperature should be 160° F.

10. Glaze with the prepared dried cherry marmalade, turn off the oven and let the loin rest inside the oven for 10–15 minutes. Take out a pork loin, slice into portions. Enjoy warm.

Nutritional Analysis

263 Calories | 22 gr Carbohydrates | 14 gr Protein | 14 gr Fat

137 mg Sodium | 154 mg Phosphorus | 275 mg Potassium

17. Slow-Cooked Bavarian Pot Roast

Makes: 12 portions

Serving size is 4 oz.

Ingredients

- Beef chuck roast, 3 pounds
- Vegetable oil, 1 tsp
- Ginger, ½ tsp, freshly ground
- Pepper, ½ tsp
- Cloves, 3, whole
- Apples, 2 cups, sliced
- Onions, ½ cup, sliced
- Apple juice, ½ cup (or water)

- Flour, 4 tbsp.
- 4 tbsp. water
- Fresh apple slices, optional garnish

Directions

1. Trim the extra fat from the beef roast. Wash and dry with a napkin. Rub the roast's top with oil, then scatter with ginger and pepper and add the whole cloves to the whole roast. Next, in a hot pan greased with oil, sear both sides of the pot roast.
2. In a crock-pot or a slow cooker, place the onions and apples. Place the pot roast and splash the roast with apple juice.
3. Cook on low heat covered for 10 to 12 hours, or around 5-6 hours, on high.
4. Extract the roast from the slow cooker. Put it aside; keep it warm, though.
5. Drain the juices from the pot roast and funnel them straight into the slow cooker. To reduce this liquid and thicken it, turn the heat to high.
6. Using flour and water, make a nice paste, then pour into the slow cooker, whisking as you mix.
7. Cover and boil until the mixture thickens. Just prior to serving, pour over the roast.

Optional: Garnish with slices of fresh apples.

Nutritional Analysis

313 Calories | 6 gr Carbohydrates | 22 gr Protein | 22 gr Total Fat

73 mg Sodium | 2020 mg Phosphorus | 373 mg Potassium

18. Herb-Roasted Chicken Breasts

Makes: 4 portions

Serving size is 4 oz.

Ingredients

- Chicken breasts, 1 pound, skinless, boneless,

- Onion, 1 medium
- Garlic, 1–2 cloves
- Herb and garlic seasoning blend, Mrs. Dash, 2 tbsp.
- Black pepper, 1 tsp freshly ground
- Olive oil, ¼ cup

Directions

Marination:

1. Chop onion and garlic and place it in a marinade bowl. Add ground pepper, seasoning, and olive oil.
2. To the marinade, add chicken breasts cover it, and refrigerate for about 4 hours or overnight.

Baking:

1. Heat the oven to 350°F.
2. Put the marinated chicken on a baking sheet covered with foil.
3. Pour the remainder marinade on the chicken breasts and bake for 20 minutes at 350°F.
4. For an additional 5 minutes, broil for browning.

Nutritional Analysis

270 Calories | 17 gr Total Fat | 3 gr Carbohydrates | 26 gr Protein

53 mg Sodium | 252 mg Phosphorus | 491 mg Potassium

19. Roasted Turkey

Makes: 8 portions plus leftovers

Serving size is 3 oz.

Ingredients

- Turkey, 12 pounds (avoid self-basting), fresh or frozen

- Fresh thyme, 4 sprigs
- Poultry seasoning, 1 tsp
- Fresh parsley, 4 sprigs
- Turkey stock, 1 cup, low-sodium (from turkey giblets)
- Fresh sage, 4 sprigs
- Unsalted butter, 1/2 cup
- Fresh rosemary, 4 sprigs

Directions

1. If it is frozen, defrost the turkey in the fridge for three days prior to roasting. Verify to assess the cooking period, plastic wrap on the turkey
2. Heat the kiln to 425 ° F.
3. Remove from the turkey's cavity the neck and giblet pocket. Wash the turkey with tap
4. Coldwater, and then, with clean paper towels, pat it dry.
5. Unstick the skin of the turkey breast and drumsticks by using your fingers. Rub the turkey flesh under the skin with poultry seasoning. Between the turkey skin and the flesh, put the parsley, rosemary, sage, and thyme sprigs.
6. In the thick part of the thigh, insert a meat thermometer, do not touch the bone.
7. Layer the turkey with oil or butter and put it breast part up on a rack in a roasting pan. With aluminum foil, cover it loosely. Bake for at least 30 minutes and then lower the heat to 325 degrees F.
8. With the giblet stock and pan juices, start basting the turkey every 15 to 20 minutes. Please take off the foil from the roasting pan within the last 30 minutes. Cook till the food thermometer registers 165 ° F for 3 to 4 hours.
9. Prior to carving, let the roasted turkey rest for 30 minutes.

Nutritional Analysis:

144 Calories | 0 gr Carbohydrates | 25 gr Protein | 4 gr Fat

57 mg Sodium | 182 mg Phosphorus | 256 mg Potassium

20. Ratatouille

Makes: 16 portions

Serving size is 1/2 cup

Ingredients:

- Zucchini squash, 2 cups
- Yellow crookneck squash, 3 cups
- Onion, 2 cups
- Eggplant, 1 medium
- Yellow bell pepper, 1
- Carrots, 2, medium
- Green bell pepper, 1
- Garlic, 4 cloves
- Red bell pepper, 1
- Olive oil, 2 tbsp.
- Tomatoes, 1 cup canned
- Fresh basil, 1 tbsp.
- Fresh oregano, 1 tbsp.
- Fresh rosemary, 1 tbsp.
- Fresh thyme, 1 tbsp.
- Fresh sage, 1 tbsp.

- Black pepper, 1 tbsp.
- Parmesan cheese, grated, 8 tbsp.

Directions:

1. Slice the onion, eggplant, squash, peppers, and carrots. Mince the cloves of garlic. Adding the Olive oil in a big saucepan, also add in the ginger, black pepper, herbs, and carrots.

2. Fry for 2 minutes, then introduce the remaining vegetables, except the tomatoes.

3. Fry well and stir regularly for 10 to 15 minutes or till the vegetables are half tender.

4. Add in parmesan cheese and tomatoes and stir well.

5. cook on low heat covered for around 1/2 hour. Serve immediately.

6. Place the leftover Ratatouille in 1 to 2 cup parts and freeze. Reheat it for A quick lunch later in the microwave.

Present the Ratatouille as a side dish or incorporate any pasta (small shells, bow ties, or elbows).

Make a full meal by serving with cooked ground turkey, beef, or Chicken.

Nutritional Analysis:

54 Calories | 3 gr Protein | 6 gr Carbohydrates | 3 gr Fat

84 mg Sodium | 302 mg Potassium | 58 mg Phosphorus

Seafood

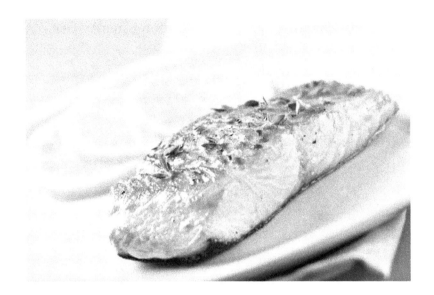

21. Baked fish

Makes: 4 portions

Serving size is 3 oz.

Ingredients

- Trout fillets, 4 3-oz (or any other baking fish)
- Black pepper, 1 ½ tsp
- Garlic powder, 1 tbsp.
- Paprika, 1 ½ tsp
- Onion, 1 small
- Green pepper, ¼ medium
- Lemon, 1 small
- Parmesan cheese, 2 tbsp.

Directions

1. Heat oven to 375°f.
2. In a greased baking tray, Place fish on an aluminum foil.

3. On both sides of fish sprinkle garlic powder, black pepper, and paprika.

4. Place Cut green peppers on fish. Also, place sliced onion rings on fish.

5. Pour lemon juice onto fish.

6. Bake for at least 30 minutes.

7. After fish has baked, scatter with parmesan cheese. Enjoy hot.

Nutritional Analysis

164 Calories | 20 gr Protein | 6 gr Fat | 8 gr Carbohydrate

86 mg Sodium | 452 mg Potassium | 252 mg Phosphorus

22. Supreme of Seafood

Makes: 6 portions

Serving size is ½ cup

Ingredients

- Crabmeat, 1 cup, cooked (boiled)
- Green pepper, 4 tbsp., chopped
- Shrimp, 1 cup, cooked (boiled)
- Green onions, 2 tbsp., chopped
- Celery, 1 cup, chopped
- Green peas, ½ cup, frozen
- Black pepper, ½ tsp
- Bread crumbs, 1 cup
- Mayonnaise, ½ cup

Directions

1. Heat oven to 375°f.

2. Mix all ingredients leaving the bread crumbs in a large bowl.

3. Put this mixture in a casserole dish greased with oil.

4. Sprinkle with bread crumbs.

5. Bake casserole for 30 minutes.

Nutritional Analysis

220 Calories | 16 gr Protein | 8 gr total Fat | 20 gr Carbohydrate

445 mg Sodium | 255 mg Potassium | 148 mg Phosphorus

23. Tuna-Noodle Skillet Dinner

Makes: 4 portions

Serving size is 4 oz. fish

Ingredients

- Vegetable cooking spray
- Fresh onion, 2 tbsp. minced
- Water, ⅔ cup
- Curry powder, ¼ tsp
- Black pepper, ¼ tsp
- Cream of mushroom soup, low sodium, 1 10 ¾-oz can, undiluted
- Cooked rotini, 2 cups hot, (, cooked without salt or fat corkscrew pasta,)
- Green peas, ½ cup frozen, thawed
- Albacore tuna, 1 9 ¼-oz low sodium, with water, drained
- Fresh parsley chopped (optional)

Directions

1. Coat with cooking spray a large nonstick skillet; position over moderate heat.

2. Add in onion; fry until soft.

3. In a bowl, mix the water, soup, pepper and, curry powder; whisk well and transfer to the skillet.

4. Add the cooked peas, rotini, and tuna; combine properly. Cook without covering, for 10 minutes over low heat, Occasional stirring.

5. If needed, garnish with parsley.

Nutritional Analysis

269 Calories | 4 gr total Fat | 38 gr Carbohydrate | 18 gr Protein

407 mg Sodium | 515 mg Potassium | 228 mg Phosphorus

24. Crab-Stuffed shrimp

Makes: 4 Portions

Serving size is 3 shrimp

Ingredients

- 6 oz. crab meat
- 1/4 cup dry bread crumbs
- 3 tbsp. unsalted butter
- 1 tsp celery
- 1 tsp parsley
- 1 tsp onion
- 1 tsp green bell pepper
- 1/4 tsp lemon juice
- 3 drops hot sauce
- 1/8 tsp garlic powder
- 1/8 tsp black pepper

- 12 jumbo shrimp, raw and shelled with tails on

Directions

1. Heat the 450 ° F oven.
2. Finely chop the parsley, celery, bell pepper, onion, and the crab meat.
3. In a bowl, combine bread crumbs, crab, 3 tbsp. of melted butter, parsley, celery, bell pepper, and onion; put aside.
4. Use a nonstick cooking spray to spray a baking dish.
5. Devein and clean the shrimp, and pat it off. (Frozen shrimps may be used -thaw before using in the recipe.)
6. Using a sharp knife to remove a 1/2"- deep pocket from the tail around the middle of the inner curved side of the shrimp, leave 1/2 "at the edge. Do not touch the shrimp's back. Using your finger to enlarge the pocket.
7. Use about 2-1/2 tbsp. per shrimp of the crab mixture. Position the crab in the shrimp pocket and spread it to fill. On a baking sheet, place the shrimp. Repeat. Have all the shrimp primed.
8. Brush the melting butter on the shrimp. For 10 to 12 minutes, bake. Don't overcook it.
9. When needed, serve with melted, unsalted butter.

Nutritional Analysis

267 Calories | 15 gr Fat | 27 gr Protein | 6 gr Carbohydrates

397 mg Sodium | 320 mg Potassium | 278 mg Phosphorus

25. Tuna Veggie Salad

Makes: 4 Portions

Serving size is 3/4 cup

Ingredients

- Bell pepper, red, 1/2 cup
- Zucchini, 1 cup
- Green bell pepper, 1/2 cup
- Green onions, 1/4 cup
- Garlic, 1 clove
- Fresh basil, 1/4 cup
- Tuna, 5 oz., can-packed in water
- Red wine vinegar, 2-1/2 tbsp.
- Olive oil, 1 tbsp.
- Black pepper, 1/8 tsp

Directions

1. Thinly slice zucchini and Dice bell peppers. Chop basil and green onions. Mince garlic.
2. Into a medium saucepan, pour 3/4 cup of water
3. Place sliced zucchini and diced bell peppers into a steamer basket and placed over a saucepan filled with water. Boil water and steam veggies for 10 minutes
4. Take off vegetables from heat, transfer to a medium serving bowl draining off any extra water.
5. Add to it green onions, basil, and tuna. Toss to mix all ingredients.
6. Combine oil, vinegar, black pepper, and garlic in a jar with a tight cover and shake it well to make the dressing.
7. Drizzle dressing over vegetable and tuna mixture and combine well.

Nutritional Analysis

88 Calories | 10 gr Protein | 4 gr Fat | 3 gr Carbohydrates

23 mg Sodium | 248 mg Potassium

26. Cilantro-Lime Cod

Make: 4 Portions

Serving size is One 3-oz fillet

Ingredients

- Mayonnaise, 1/2 cup
- Lime juice, 2 tbsp.
- Fresh cilantro, 1/2 cup
- Cod fillets, 1 pound

Directions

1. Combine mayonnaise, lime juice, and chopped cilantro in a medium bowl. Separate 1/4 cup of the sauce into a small bowl and put aside to serve with the fish.
2. Coat fish with remainder mayonnaise mixture.
3. With a nonstick cooking spray, spray a large skillet and heat on medium-high heat. Put cod fillets in it and cook both sides turning once, until fish is moist but firm for about 8 minutes.
4. Serve with remainder cilantro-lime sauce.

Nutritional Analysis

292 Calories | 23 gr Fat | 20 gr Protein | 1 gr Carbohydrates

228 mg Sodium | 237 mg Potassium | 128 mg Phosphorus

27. Grilled Trout

Makes: 8 Portions

Serving size is 3 oz.

Ingredients

- 2 pounds rainbow trout fillets
- 1 tbsp. cooking oil
- 1/2 tsp salt
- 1 tsp salt-free lemon pepper
- 1/2 tsp paprika

Directions

1. Heat grill on high heat.
2. Spray or brush the trout fillets lightly with oil on all sides. Mix the spices in a small bowl. Rub thoroughly on the fillets.
3. Put the seasoned trout directly on the heated grill, fillet side down. Grill for 4 minutes. Brush or spray the skin with oil lightly. Turn over the fillets and cook till the fish flakes with a fork easily, around 3 to 5 minutes.

Nutritional Analysis

161 Calories | 8 gr Fat | 21 gr Protein | 0 gr Carbohydrates

169 mg Sodium | 385 mg Potassium | 227 mg Phosphorus

28. Crunchy Oven-Fried Catfish

Makes: 4 Portions

Serving size is 3 oz.

Ingredients

- Egg white, 1
- All-purpose flour, 1/2 cup
- Cornmeal, 1/4 cup
- Catfish fillets, 1 pound

- Bread crumbs, panko, 1/4 cup
- Cajun seasoning, salt-free, 1 tsp

Directions

1. Preheat oven to 450° F.
2. Spray with nonstick cooking spray on the top of a flat, nonstick baking tray.
3. In a shallow bowl, beat the egg whites till very soft peaks form. Try not to over-beat.
4. Sprinkle flour on a wax paper sheet.
5. Combine the panko, cornmeal, and Cajun seasoning on another wax paper sheet.
6. Divide catfish fillet into a total of four portions. Submerge the fish into the flour and shake off extra.
7. Then dip in the whisked egg white.
8. And roll in the mixture of cornmeal.
9. Place coated fish on the baking tray, and go over steps 6 to 9 with all fillets.
10. with cooking spray, spray-on tops of the fish fillets and bake for about 10 to 12 minutes, till the fish fillets are browned and sizzling. Take out the pan from the oven and turn the fish to the other side.
11. Put back in the oven and more bake for 5 minutes until fillets are crisp and browned.

Nutritional Analysis

250 Calories | 10 gr Fat | 22 gr Protein | 19 gr Carbohydrates

124 mg Sodium | 401 mg Potassium | 262 mg Phosphorus

29. Linguine with Garlic and Shrimp

Make: 6 Portions

Serving size is 1-1/2 cups

Ingredients

- Raw shrimp, 3/4 pound
- Flat-leaf parsley, 1 cup
- Water, 2-1/2 quarts
- Linguine, uncooked, 12 oz.
- Olive oil, 2 tbsp.
- Garlic, 2 heads whole
- Lemon juice, 1 tbsp.
- Black pepper, 1/4 tsp

Directions

1. Clean and Peel shrimp. Chop the parsley.
2. In a large pot, boil water. Include pasta and boil until tender or for 10 minutes.
3. When pasta is cooking, separate the garlic cloves with skin on. Fry cloves in a pan on medium heat, stirring constantly. When it becomes soft to touch and darkens, the garlic is ready. Skin will remove easily. Remove from pan and peel the skin.
4. In a sauté pan, heat olive oil, and put back peeled garlic in the pan. Fry garlic till golden.
5. Add shrimp and parsley and cook for 1 to 2 minutes till shrimp becomes pink.
6. Draining pasta, reserve 1 cup of liquid. Add drained pasta to the frying pan with garlic and shrimp. Combine all ingredients and add the reserved liquid to it.
7. Add black pepper and lemon juice. Stir and serve.

Nutritional Analysis

322 Calories | 6 gr Fat | 20 gr Protein | 47 gr Carbohydrates

106 mg Sodium | 298 mg Potassium | 220 mg Phosphorus

30. Jambalaya

Makes: 12 Portions

Serving size is 1 cup

Ingredients

- Onion, 2 cups
- Bell pepper, 1 cup
- Garlic cloves, 2
- Raw shrimp, 2 pounds
- Converted (parboiled) white rice, uncooked, 2 cups
- Black pepper, ½ tsp
- Canned low-sodium tomato sauce, 8 oz.
- Low-sodium beef broth, 2 cups
- Butter or trans-fat free margarine, ½ cup

Directions

1. Heat the oven to 350° F.
2. Chop the garlic, onion, and bell pepper. Devein and Peel the shrimp.
3. Combine all the given ingredients in a big bowl, leaving butter.
4. Into a 9" x 13" baking dish, pour the mixture and spread evenly.
5. Chop the butter into small pieces and place them on top of the mixture.
6. Cover tray with foil.
7. For 1 hour and 15 minutes, bake. Enjoy hot.

Nutritional Analysis

294 Calories | 10 gr Fat | 20 gr Protein | 31 gr Carbohydrates

186 mg Sodium | 300 mg Potassium | 197 mg Phosphorus

Poultry

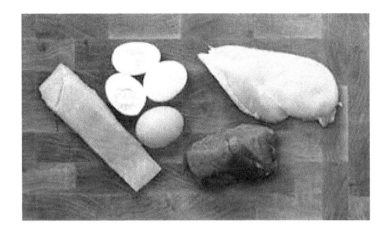

31. Turkey & Noodles

Makes: 6 portions

Serving size is 1 cup

Ingredients

- Elbow macaroni, 2 cups dry
- Vegetable, 1 tbsp. (or olive oil)
- Lean ground turkey, 2 pounds fresh
- Green onions, ½ cup, chopped
- Green pepper, ½ cup, chopped
- Regular tomatoes, 1 14-oz can, diced
- Italian seasoning, 1 tbsp.
- Black pepper, 1 tsp

Directions

1. Start by boiling water in a large boiler, add macaroni. Let boil until desired tenderness or for 5 minutes. Drain macaroni and put aside.
2. In a large skillet, heat veg. Oil on medium heat. In heated oil, add ground turkey, stirring

occasionally, and cook until done.

3. Add diced tomatoes, green peppers, onions, black pepper, Italian seasoning, and cooked macaroni. Combine well.

4. Cover and cook for further 5 minutes. Serve warm.

Nutritional Analysis

273 Calories | 33 gr Protein | 7 gr total Fat | 22 gr Carbohydrates

188 mg Sodium | 533 mg Potassium | 296 mg Phosphorus

32. Barbecue Cups

Makes: 10 servings

Serving size is 1 biscuit

Ingredients

- Ground turkey, ¾ pounds lean
- Spicy barbecue sauce, ½ cup
- Onion flakes, 2 tsp
- Garlic powder, dash
- Refrigerator biscuits, low-fat, 1 10-oz package

Directions

1. In a nonstick skillet, cook turkey until brown.
2. Add garlic powder, barbecue sauce, and onion flakes. Combine well.
3. Grease muffin tins, flatten one biscuit, and push into muffin tin one at a time.
4. Add beef mixture with a spoon into each biscuit cup's center.
5. Bake for 10 to 12 minutes at 400°f.

Nutritional Analysis

134 Calories | 7 gr Protein | 5 gr total Fat | 13 gr Carbohydrate

342 mg Sodium | 151 mg Potassium | 152 mg Phosphorus

33. Crispy Oven Fried Chicken

Makes: 8 pieces

Serving size is 3 or 4-ozs

Ingredients

- Fryer chicken, 2 ½ pounds, (cut as desired)
- Lemon juice, 1 tablespoon
- All-purpose flour, 1 cup
- Black pepper, 1 tsp
- Corn flakes, 1 cup, crushed
- Poultry seasoning, ¼ tsp
- Vegetable oil, 4 tbsp.

Directions

1. Heat oven to 400°F.
2. Rinse chicken pieces thoroughly and dry with a kitchen towel; massage with lemon juice.
3. Mix flour, corn flakes, poultry seasoning, and black pepper in a small bag. Shake thoroughly.
4. Grease a shallow baking tray (about "deep) with vegetable oil.
5. Put the chicken in the bag of flour and seasoning mixture; put in the large pieces first. Shake thoroughly.
6. Put the coated chicken in the greased pan.
7. Bake for 20-30 minutes on each side until brown.

Nutritional Analysis

280 Calories | 15 gr Protein | 18 gr total Fat | 15 gr Carbohydrate

74 mg Sodium | 150 mg Potassium | 120 mg Phosphorus

34. Jalepeno Pepper Chicken

Makes: 8 servings

Serving size is 3-oz

Ingredients

- Vegetable oil, 3 tbsp.
- Chicken, cut up, 2-3 pounds (skin and fat removed)
- Onion, 1, sliced into rings
- Chicken bouillon, low-sodium, 1 ½ cups
- Ground nutmeg, ½ tsp
- Black pepper, ¼ tsp
- Jalapeño peppers, 2 tsp, fresh, chopped finely, and seeded

Directions

1. Put a big skillet on medium-high heat with oil and cook the chicken pieces till brown. Put aside, keep it warm.
2. Sauté onion rings in hot oil. Put in bouillon and bring it to a boil, stirring frequently.
3. Put chicken back in pan; add black pepper and nutmeg. Top with lid and simmer until chicken is soft or for 35 minutes.
4. Mix in jalapeño peppers, and cook on low for another minute.

Nutritional Analysis

143 Calories | 17 gr Protein | 7 gr total Fat | 2 gr Carbohydrate

45 mg Sodium | 160 mg Potassium

35. Stuffed Green Peppers

Make: 6 servings

Serving size is 1 stuffed pepper

Ingredients

- Vegetable oil, 2 tbsp.
- Turkey, ½ pound ground and lean (or chicken)
- Onions, ¼ cup, chopped
- Celery, ¼ cup, chopped
- Lemon juice, 2 tbsp.
- Celery seed, 1 tbsp.
- Italian seasoning, 2 tbsp.
- Black pepper, 1 tsp
- Sugar, ½ tsp
- Cooked rice, 1 ½ cups
- Paprika
- Green peppers, 6 smalls, seeded with tops removed

Directions

1. Heat oven to 325°F.
2. In a saucepan, heat oil.
3. Add onions, ground meat, and celery; cook till meat is good and brown.
4. Include all ingredients in a saucepan, leaving paprika and green peppers. Mix together, take off from the heat.
5. Fill the peppers with cooked mixture. Put foil over it or put in a baking dish and cover.
6. Bake for around 30 minutes. Take out and season with paprika.

Nutritional Analysis

131 Calories | 9 gr Protein | 4 gr total Fat | 15 gr Carbohydrate

36 mg Sodium | 160 mg Potassium | 83 mg Phosphorus

---

36. Easy Chicken and Pasta Dinner

Makes: 2 Portions

Serving size is 1 cup pasta

Ingredients

- Chicken, 2-1/2 oz.
- Vegetables, 2/3 cup
- 1/2 cup red bell pepper
- 1 cup zucchini
- 1 tablespoon olive oil
- 2 cups cooked pasta, any shape
- 5 oz. cooked chicken breast
- 3 tbsp. low-sodium Italian dressing

Directions

1. Slice bell pepper and zucchini.
2. Take a nonstick pan, heat the olive oil, and sauté peppers and zucchini until crispy tender. Take out in a plate.
3. Cut meat into strips.
4. Heat chicken strips and cooked pasta in the microwave one by one.
5. Mix pasta with dressing. Dish out with chicken strips and sautéed vegetables.

If you require a higher or lower protein diet, adjust the portion of chicken in this dish.

Nutritional Analysis:

400 Calories | 11 gr Fat | 30 gr Protein | 45 gr Carbohydrates

328 mg Sodium | 270 mg Phosphorus | 455 mg Potassium

37. Chicken Nuggets with Honey Mustard Dipping Sauce

Makes: 12 Portions

Serving size is 3 nuggets plus 1 tablespoon sauce

Ingredients

- Yellow mustard, 1 tablespoon
- Mayonnaise, 1/2 cup
- Honey, 1/3 cup
- Worcestershire sauce, 2 tsp
- Chicken breasts, 1 pound, boneless
- Low-fat milk, 1%, 2 tbsp.
- Cornflakes, 3 cups
- Egg, 1 large

Directions

1. In a small bowl, Stir the mayonnaise, mustard, Worcestershire sauce, and honey together. Chill the sauce in a Refrigerator till the nuggets are done, then use it as a dipping sauce.

2. Heat the oven to 400° F.

3. Slice the breast pieces into 36 same-sized pieces.

4. Squash the cornflakes and transfer the crumbs into a big zip-lock bag.

5. Take a small mixing bowl, beat the egg, and then mix it with milk. Dunk the small chicken pieces in the whisked egg, then put in a Ziplock bag and shake to coat with the cornflake crumbs.

6. on the baking tray sprayed with nonstick cooking spray, Put the nuggets and bake for 15

minutes or until tender.

Nutritional Analysis:

164 Calories | 8 gr Fat | 9 gr Protein | 14 gr Carbohydrates

157 mg Sodium | 99 mg Potassium | 70 mg Phosphorus

---

38. Indian Chicken Curry

Makes: around 12 pieces

Serving size is two small drumsticks

Ingredients

- Tomato, 1 medium
- Onions, 2, medium
- Garlic, 2 cloves
- Ginger root, 1" cube
- Chicken drumsticks, small, 1-1/2 pounds
- Vegetable oil, 5 tbsp.
- Whole cumin seeds, 3/4 tsp
- Cinnamon stick, 1
- Bay leaves, 2
- Whole peppercorns, 1/4 tsp
- Salt, 3/4 tsp
- Cayenne pepper, 1-1/2 tsp
- Garam masala, 1/2 tsp

Directions

1. Peel the tomato and chop. Mince the garlic, ginger root, and onion. Take off and discard the skin from the chicken.

2. heat the oil in a wide, large pot, on medium-high flame. Add to it the cumin seeds, bay leaves, cinnamon stick, and peppercorns. Stirring once.

3. Also, add the garlic, ginger, and onion. Stir these ingredients till the onion gets brown specks.

4. To it, add the chicken, tomato, cayenne pepper, salt, and ¼ cup water. Stir and take to a boil.

5. Put on the lid on the pot tightly, reduce the heat, and simmer for about 25 minutes on low heat or till the chicken is soft and tender. Stirring in between the cooking period.

6. Take off the cover and increase heat to medium. Season with garam masala and stirring gently cook to decrease the liquid for about 5 minutes.

Nutritional Analysis:

269 Calories | 18 gr Fat | 21 gr Protein | 6 gr Carbohydrates

350 mg Sodium | 286 mg Potassium | 139 mg Phosphorus

39. Chicken and Summer Vegetable Kebabs

Makes: 6 Portions

Serving size is 1 large kebab or 2 small kebabs.

Ingredients

- Olive oil, 2 tbsp.
- Peach jam, 1 tablespoon
- Lemon juice, 2 tbsp.
- Herb seasoning blend, 1 tsp
- Salt, 1/4 tsp
- Chicken thighs, boneless, skinless, 1 pound
- Zucchini, 1 medium
- Summer squash, 1 medium, yellow
- Bell pepper, 1 red

- Onion, 1 medium

Directions

1. Into a small microwave-safe bowl, measure the peach jam to make the marinade by heating for 10 to 15 seconds in the microwave to liquefy. Include the herb seasoning olive oil, lemon juice, and salt. Mix well until blended.

2. Wash the chicken thighs and with a paper towel, pat dry. Chop each boneless thigh into 4 pieces and put in a zip-lock bag.

3. Add half of the marinade to the boneless pieces. (remaining half of marinade to be used on the veggies.) Close the zip-lock bag and put it in the fridge to marinate.

4. Slice the veggies into small-sized pieces to make kebabs. Put them in a container and add the remaining marinade. Mix to coat the veggies.

5. Thread the chicken pieces and vegetables onto skewers (8 small or 4 large skewers).

6. On a Heated medium grill, place the skewers, and cook with cover for 12 to 15 minutes. To cook evenly, Turn the skewers frequently.

Nutritional Analysis:

284 Calories | 16 gr Fat | 24 gr Protein | 10 gr Carbohydrates

215 mg Sodium | 456 mg Potassium | 194 mg Phosphorus

40. Easy Turkey Sloppy Joes

Makes: 6 Portions

Serving size is 1/6 recipe on 1 bun.

Ingredients

- Red onion, 1/2 cup
- Ground turkey, 7% fat, 1-1/2 pounds
- Bell pepper green, 1/2 cup
- Chicken grilling seasoning blend, 1 tbsp.

- Brown sugar, 2 tbsp.
- Worcestershire sauce, 1 tbsp.
- Tomato sauce, 1 cup, low-sodium
- Hamburger buns, 6

Directions

1. Chop the bell pepper and onion.
2. in a large skillet, Place the vegetables with ground turkey and cook on medium-high till turkey is thoroughly cooked. Do not drain the liquid.
3. Mix together the brown sugar, grilling seasoning, tomato sauce, and Worcestershire sauce in a small bowl.
4. Add the above sauce to the meat mixture. Lower heat and simmer for 10 minutes.
5. Split the turkey mix into 6 parts and serve on burger buns.

Nutritional Analysis:

290 Calories | 9 gr Fat | 24 gr Protein | 28 gr Carbohydrates

288 mg Sodium | 237 mg Phosphorus | 513 mg Potassium

Meat

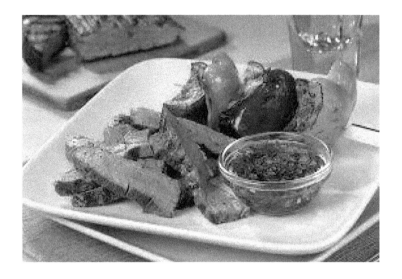

41. Chili Rice with Beef

Makes: 4 portions

Serving size is 1 cup

Ingredients

- Vegetable oil, 2 tbsp.
- Ground beef, 1 pound, lean
- Onion, 1 cup, chopped
- Rice, 2 cups, cooked
- Chili con carne seasoning powder, 1 ½ tsp
- Black pepper, ⅛ tsp
- Sage, ½ tsp

Directions

1. In a pan, heat oil; include beef and onion. Fry, frequently stirring until brown.
2. Include cooked rice and add seasoning. Combine together.
3. Take off from the heat. With a lid, cover and put aside for 10-14 minutes, then serve.

Nutritional Analysis

360 Calories | 23 gr Protein | 14 gr total Fat | 26 gr Carbohydrate

78 mg Sodium | 427 mg Potassium | 233 mg Phosphorus

42. Parsley Burger

Makes: 4 portions

Serving size is 1 patty, 3-ozs

Ingredients

- Ground beef, lean, 1 pound
- Black pepper, ¼ tsp
- Lemon juice, 1 tbsp.
- Ground thyme, ¼ tsp
- Parsley flakes, 1 tbsp.
- Oregano, ¼ tsp

Directions

1. Combine all the ingredients finely.
2. Make into 4 small equal-sized patties around ¾" thick.
3. Put on a lightly oiled skillet or a pan.
4. Broil for about 3" away from the heat, turning once for 10 to 15 minutes.

Nutritional Analysis

171 Calories | 20 gr Protein | 10 gr total Fat | 0 gr Carbohydrate

108 mg Sodium | 289 mg Potassium | 180 mg Phosphorus

43. Swedish Meatballs

Makes: 35 meatballs

Serving size is 2 meatballs

Ingredients

For meatballs

- Ground beef, lean, 1 pound
- Onions, ¼ cup, finely chopped
- Lemon juice, 1 tbsp.
- Poultry seasoning, 1 tsp (without salt)
- Black pepper, 1 tsp
- Italian seasoning, 1 tsp
- Dry mustard, ¼ tsp
- Granulated sugar, 1 tsp
- ¾ tsp onion powder
- Tabasco sauce, 1 tsp

Directions for meatballs

1. Heat oven to 425°f.
2. Combine all ingredients well together.
3. Make meatballs by taking one tbsp. mixture for every meatball.
4. Put meatballs in a baking tray and bake for at least 20 minutes or till well done. Prepare the sauce (recipe below).
5. Take out meatballs from the oven and drizzle with sauce. Keep hot until ready to serve.

For sauce

- Vegetable oil, ¼ cup
- All-purpose flour, 2 tbsp.
- Onion powder, 1 tsp
- Vinegar, 2 tsp
- Tabasco sauce, 1 tsp
- Sugar, 2 tsp
- Water, 2-3 cups

Directions for sauce

6. Combine flour and oil in a saucepan on medium heat; keep stirring till golden brown. Take off from the heat. Add vinegar, sugar, onion powder, Tabasco sauce, and water.

7. Put back on the heat and keep on mixing until the desired thickness.

Nutritional Analysis

76 Calories | 5 gr Protein | 6 gr total Fat | 2 gr Carbohydrate

31 mg Sodium | 70 mg Potassium | 44 mg Phosphorus

44. Open-Faced Steak & Onion Sandwich

Makes: 2 portions

Serving size is 1 sandwich

Ingredients

- Chopped steaks, 4, (4-ozs each)
- Lemon juice, 1 tbsp.
- Italian seasoning, 1 tbsp.
- Black pepper, 1 tbsp.
- Vegetable oil, 1 tbsp.

- Onion, 1 medium, sliced into rings
- Herbed bread, 4 slices

Directions

1. Season meat with black pepper, Italian seasoning, and lemon juice.
2. In a sauté pan, heat oil on medium heat.
3. Cook seasoned steaks till browned on both sides and tender. Remove from pan and drain on paper.
4. Reduce heat; put in the onion and sauté till onions are soft.
5. Dish up open-faced topped with onion rings on herbed bread.

Nutritional Analysis

345 Calories | 14 gr Protein | 21 gr total Fat | 26 gr Carbohydrate

247 mg Sodium | 200 mg Potassium | 115 mg Phosphorus

45. Homemade Pan Sausage

Makes: 12 portions

Serving size is 1 patty

Ingredients

- Cooking spray
- Ground pork, 1 pound, fresh lean (or beef)
- Granulated sugar, 2 tsp
- Ground black pepper, 1 tsp
- Ground sage, 2 tsp
- Ground red pepper, ½ tsp
- Basil, 1 tsp (optional)

Directions

1. Combine all ingredients very well, to make sausage.
2. To make into a patty, take 2 tbsp. of meat mixture and form patties.
3. broil or Pan fry until cooked thoroughly.

Nutritional Analysis

22 Calories | 6 gr Protein | 7 gr total Fat | 1 gr Carbohydrate

22 mg Sodium | 87 mg Potassium | 53 mg Phosphorus

46. Spicy Beef Stir-Fry

Makes: 4 portions

Serving size is 1 cup

Ingredients

- Cornstarch, 2 Tbsp., separated
- Sesame oil, ¼ tsp
- Sugar, ½ tsp
- Water, 2 Tbsp., separated
- Egg, 1 large, beaten
- Canola oil, 3 Tbsp., separated
- Beef round tip, 12 oz., sliced
- Bell pepper, 1 green, sliced
- Onions, 1 cup, sliced
- Red chili pepper, ¼ tsp, ground (or to taste)
- Sherry, 1 tbsp.
- Soy sauce, 2 tsp, reduced-sodium
- Parsley (optional garnish)

Directions

1. In a big bowl, mix 1 tbsp. cornstarch, 1 large egg, 1 tbsp. canola oil, 1 tbsp. water, and include the beef. Keep aside for 20 minutes.

2. In another bowl, mix the remaining water and cornstarch. Put aside.

3. In a skillet, heat the remainder 2 tbsp. of oil and include the marinated meat mix. Cook till the meat browns.

4. In it, add the onion, green bell peppers, and chili pepper. Drizzle with sherry, and stir-fry all of it for a minute. Add in sesame oil, sugar, and soy sauce.

5. Pour in cornstarch and water mixture. Stir till it thickens and serve.

Nutritional Analysis

261 Calories | 15 gr total Fat | 10 gr Carbohydrates | 21 gr Protein

169 mg Sodium | 167mg Phosphorus | 313mg Potassium

47. Pasta with Cheesy Meat Sauce

Makes: 6 portions

Serving size is 8 oz.

Ingredients

- Pasta, large-shaped, ½ box
- Ground beef, 1 pound
- Onions, ½ cup, diced
- Onion flakes, 1 tbsp.
- Beef stock, 1½ cups, reduced-sodium
- Beef bouillon, 1 tbsp., no salt added
- Tomato sauce, 1 tbsp., no salt added
- Pepper jack or Monterey cheese, ¾ cup shredded

- Cream cheese, 8 oz., softened
- Italian seasoning, ½ tsp
- Black pepper, ½ tsp, ground
- Worcestershire sauce, 2 tbsp., reduced-sodium

Directions

1. Boil pasta as given directions on the box.
2. Cook ground beef in a large fry pan. Add onion flakes and onions, fry till the meat is good and brown.
3. Drain the pasta and add bouillon, stock, and tomato sauce to the browned meat.
4. Cook the above until it starts to simmer, stirring often. Add cooked pasta, take off heat, mix in shredded cheese, softened cream cheese, and seasonings (black pepper, Italian seasoning, and Worcestershire sauce).
5. Mix pasta and meat mixture till cheese is throughout melted.

Nutritional Analysis

502 Calories | 30gr total Fat | 35gr Carbohydrates | 23gr Protein

401 mg Sodium | 278 mg Phosphorus | 549 mg Potassium

48. Hawaiian-Style Slow-Cooked Pulled Pork

Makes: 16 portions

Serving size is 4 oz.

Ingredients

- Pork roast, 4 pounds
- Black pepper, ½ tsp, freshly ground
- Paprika, ½ tsp
- Onion powder, 1 tsp

- Garlic powder, ½ tsp
- Liquid smoke, 2 tbsp.
- Pickled or radishes red onions (optional garnish) *
- 4 radishes or 1 red onion, white vinegar ⅓ cup, and sugar ¼ tsp.

Directions

1. In a small container, mix paprika, black pepper, garlic powder, and onion.
2. Apply the seasoning mix on all sides of the pork. Put the pork into a crock-pot or a slow cooker. Sprinkle in liquid smoke.
3. Include enough water in the crock-pot or slow cooker to measure ¼–½" deep. For 4–5 hours, Cook on high.
4. Remove pork from cooker and, using two forks, shred meat.

Nutritional Analysis

285 Calories | 21gr total Fat | 1 gr Carbohydrates | 20gr Protein

54 mg Sodium | 230mg Phosphorus | 380 mg Potassium

Vegetables

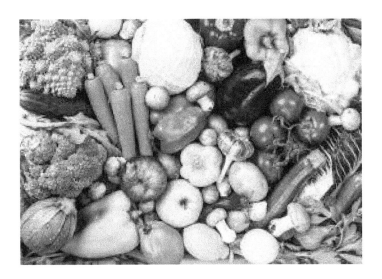

49. Coleslaw

Makes: 4 portions

Serving size is ½ cup

Ingredients

- Cabbage, 1 cup, shredded
- Green pepper, 2 tbsp., chopped
- Onion, ¼ cup, chopped
- Carrots, ¼ cup, shredded
- Mayonnaise, ¼ cup
- Vinegar, 2 tbsp.
- Sugar, 1 tbsp.
- Black pepper, ½ tsp
- Dill weeds, ⅛ tsp (optional)
- Celery seed, ½ tsp (optional)

Directions

1. Mix all vegetables.

2. Whisk together mayonnaise, seasonings, and vinegar.

3. Dump over vegetables and mix.

Nutritional Analysis

127 Calories | 0 gr Protein | 11 gr total Fat | 6 gr Carbohydrate

81 mg Sodium | 76 mg Potassium | 14 mg Phosphorus

---

50. Vegetables & Rice

Makes: 6 servings

Serving size is ½ cup

Ingredients

- Rice, cooked, 2 ½ cups, salt-free
- Green peas, frozen, 1 10-oz package, cooked and drained
- Onion, 1 medium, chopped
- Margarine, ¼ cup, unsalted
- Lemon juice, 1 tbsp.
- Thyme, ½ tsp
- Liquid smoke, 2 tbsp. (optional)

Directions

1. Fry chopped onion until tender in margarine.

2. Add green peas, cooked rice, thyme, liquid smoke, and lemon juice.

3. Cook and occasionally stir for 5 minutes.

Nutritional Analysis

194 Calories | 4 gr Protein | 8 gr total Fat | 26 gr Carbohydrate

32 mg Sodium | 99 mg Potassium | 67 mg Phosphorus

51. Favorite Green Beans

Makes: 6 servings

Serving size is ½ cup

Ingredients

- Green beans, whole, 2 cans, drained and rinsed
- Onion, 1 small, chopped
- Fresh mushrooms, ½ cup, sliced
- Paprika, 1 tsp
- Black pepper, coarse, ¼ tsp
- Top cracker crumbs, 1 ½ cups, unsalted
- Margarine, 4 tbsp., unsalted

Directions

1. Heat oven to 350°F.

2. Combine green beans, mushrooms, onion, black pepper, and paprika.

3. Put in a baking casserole dish that is greased.

4. Sprinkle bean mixture with cracker crumbs and drizzle margarine.

5. Bake for about 30-35 minutes.

Nutritional Analysis

137 Calories | 2 gr Protein | 9 gr total Fat | 14 gr Carbohydrate

77 mg Sodium | 214 mg Potassium | 38 mg Phosphorus

52. Roasted Red Pepper with Basil, Vegan Provolone Cheese Sandwiches

Makes: 2 Portions

Serving size is 1 sandwich

Ingredients

- Red bell peppers, 2 medium
- Sandwich rolls, 2, whole-grain
- Olive oil, 1 tbsp.
- Daiya cheese, provolone-style, 4 slices
- Vegan cheese, 8
- Basil leaves, fresh

Directions

1. Wash and dry red peppers with a paper towel. Ignite two burners on the medium of the stove. Place each pepper, using tongs, on the burners. As one side starts to appear black, using tongs, turn the peppers. Keep turning and cooking until all the peppers are blackened. It will take about 5- 7 minutes.

2. Place the peppers, using tongs, in a paper bag, cover. Put aside for 5 to 8 minutes.

3. In the meantime, slit both rolls lengthwise in half.

4. In a small bowl, pour olive oil. Brush oil in the inside of each sandwich roll.

5. Arrange Daiya cheese (2 slices) on the bottom half of each roll. Place in a toaster oven. Toast till cheese begins to melt. Take out rolls from the toaster and put aside.

6. Take out the red peppers from the bag. Get rid of the outer blackened skin of the pepper with your fingers.

7. Remove the pepper's stem and slit open peppers to discard the seeds and any extra water with a paper sheet. Slice the peppers in half.

8. To make a sandwich, arrange two halved peppers on each roll half, scatter fresh basil leaves, and top with the other half roll.

Nutritional Analysis

502 Calories | 22gr Fat | 11gr Protein | 65gr Carbohydrates

665 mg Sodium | 528mg Potassium | 260 mg Phosphorus

53. Vegetarian Egg Fried Rice

Makes: 6 Portions

Serving size is 1 cup

Ingredients

- Garlic, 2 cloves
- Fresh ginger, 1 tbsp
- Medium carrots, 2
- Yellow onion, 1 cup
- Extra-firm tofu, 1 cup
- Cilantro, ½ cup
- Green onions, 2
- Large eggs, 6
- Canola oil, 3 tbsp
- Green peas, ½ cup
- Dry mustard, ¼ tsp
- Rice, 4 cups, cooked
- Soy sauce, reduced-sodium, 1 tbsp

Directions

1. Mince the ginger root and garlic. Dice the tofu and yellow onion. Slice the carrots. Chop the green onions and cilantro.

2. Whisk the eggs, and in a skillet, cook like an omelet. break cooked eggs into small pieces and put aside.

3. In a skillet, on medium flame, heat the oil. Stir in the ginger, garlic, yellow onion, carrots, peas, tofu, and dry mustard.

4. As carrots get soft, add the chopped eggs, rice, and soy sauce. Combine and take off from the heat.

5. Scatter with green onions and cilantro and serve.

Nutritional Analysis

342 Calories | 15gr Protein | 37gr Carbohydrates | 15gr Fat

238 mg Sodium | 230 mg Phosphorus | 350mg Potassium

54. Spicy Chickpeas (Chana Masala)

Makes: 4 Portions

Serving size is 1-1/4 cups

Ingredients

- Medium onion, 1
- Canned chickpeas, 30 oz
- Canola oil, 2 tbsp
- Canned, tomatoes, 8 oz, diced, unsalted
- Chili powder, 1 tsp
- Fresh ginger, 1 tbsp
- Coriander powder, 1 tsp
- Garlic, 3 cloves

- Garam masala, 1 tsp
- Fresh cilantro, ¼ cup
- Ground turmeric, 1 tsp
- Lemon wedges, 4

Directions

1. Chop the cilantro and onion; mince the ginger and garlic. Pour out and rinse the canned chickpeas in a big skillet, heat the oil and sauté onion, ginger, and garlic for 3 minutes.
2. Include the tomatoes and for another 3 to 4 minutes to keep cooking.
3. Add the garam masala, coriander powder, chili powder, and turmeric; Combine well and cook for another 1 minute.
4. Put in the chickpeas and also 1/2 cup of water. Let cook on low flame for around 10 to 15 minutes.
5. Garnish with lemon wedge and cilantro. Serve with rice, naan bread; if desired,

Nutritional Analysis

400 Calories | 13gr Fat | 16gr Protein | 55gr Carbohydrates

480 mg Sodium | 455 mg Potassium | 200 mg Phosphorus

55. Breakfast Burrito

Makes: 2 Portions

Serving size is 1 burrito.

Ingredients

- Cooking spray, nonstick
- Eggs, 4
- Green chiles, 3 tbsp, diced
- Ground cumin, 1/4 tsp

- Hot pepper sauce, 1/2 tsp
- Flour tortillas, 2, burrito size

Directions

1. With a cooking spray, grease a medium-size pan and heat on medium heat.
2. Beat eggs in a bowl with green chiles, hot sauce, and cumin. Pour beaten eggs into a hot skillet and fry and stir for 1 to 2 minutes till eggs are cooked.
3. In a separate skillet, heat tortillas on medium heat or place in microwave for 20 seconds. Put half of the egg mixture on each cooked tortilla and roll it up burrito style.

Nutritional Analysis

366 Calories | 18gr Fat | 18gr Protein | 22 gr Carbohydrates

594 mg Sodium | 245 mg Potassium | 300 mg Phosphorus

56. Garlicky Penne Pasta with Asparagus

Makes: 6 portions

Serving size is 1 cup

Ingredients

- Olive oil, 2 tbsp
- Garlic, 6 cloves
- Butter, 2 tbsp
- Red pepper, 1/8 tsp, flakes
- Asparagus, 1 pound
- Tabasco, 1/4 tsp, hot sauce
- Lemon juice, 2 tsp
- Black pepper, 1/2 tsp
- Penne pasta, whole wheat, 8 oz, uncooked

- Parmesan cheese, ¼ cup shredded

Directions

1. Boil pasta as per instructions, but 2without salt.
2. Chop 2-inch pieces of all asparagus. Finely chop garlic.
3. On medium flame, heat butter and olive oil in a medium skillet. Add red pepper flakes and garlic and for 2-3 minutes sauté.
4. Add in it asparagus, lemon juice, Tabasco sauce, and black pepper and cook for another 6 minutes until crisp and tender.
5. Empty pasta in a strainer and add to a bowl. Include asparagus and mix till well coated.
6. Sprinkle with shredded cheese
7. Serve immediately.

Nutritional Analysis

258 Calories | 10 gr Fat | 9 gr Protein | 33 gr Carbohydrates

93 mg Sodium | 168 mg Phosphorus | 258 mg Potassium

57. Vegetarian Pizza

Makes: 8 Portions (two 12 inches, pizzas)

Serving size is 1/4 of pizza

Ingredients

- Red onion, 1/2 cup
- Bell pepper, green, 1/2 cup
- Mushroom pieces, 1/3 cup
- Pineapple, 1/2 cup, tidbits

- Mozzarella, part-skim cheese, 1/2 cup, shredded
- Parmesan cheese, 2 tbsps., grated
- Roasted pepper tomato sauce, 1 cup
- Readymade pizza dough (or make at home)

Directions

1. Dice and chop onion and bell pepper.

2. Heat oven to 425° F.

3. Prepare dough if not using readymade.

3. Roll out dough to prepare two 12" pizza crusts.

4. Cover each pizza with 1/2 cup Tomato Sauce.

5. Top with mushrooms, red onion, pineapple, and bell pepper.

6. Top with Parmesan and mozzarella cheeses.

7. Put in the oven for around 12-16 minutes till the top is browned and bubbly.

Nutritional Analysis

289 Calories | 12 gr Fat | 8gr Protein | 37gr Carbohydrates

165 mg Sodium | 111 mg Phosphorus | 210 mg Potassium

58. Tempeh Pita Sandwiches

Makes: 4 Portion

Serving size is 3 slices tempeh with 1/2 pita

Ingredients

- Tempeh, 8 oz
- Sesame oil, 2 tbsp
- Onion, 1 small
- Balsamic vinegar, 2 tbsp

- Bell pepper, red, 1
- Mushrooms, 1/2 cup
- Pita bread, 2 pieces, 6-inch size
- Mayonnaise, 4 tsp

Directions

1. Slice tempeh into 12 pieces. Thinly slice bell pepper, mushrooms and, onion.
2. Heat 1 tbsp oil of sesame in a big skillet on medium heat. Put in sliced tempeh and fry for 3 to 4 minutes on each side until brown. Cook for one minute after adding balsamic vinegar; turn them over and cook for an added minute. Take out tempeh from skillet.
3. Pour in remainder sesame oil in skillet and heat on medium heat. Put in the bell pepper, onion, and mushrooms and sauté until tender.
4. Split pita in half and open up to form an opening. Spread 1 tsp mayonnaise in each half. Include 1/4 of the veggie mix and 3 slices of tempeh to each pita half. Immediately Serve.

Nutritional Analysis

313 Calories | 17 gr Fat | 15 gr Protein | 25 gr Carbohydrates

187 mg Sodium | 208 mg Phosphorus | 437 mg Potassium

59. Veggie Strata

Makes: 9 Portions

Serving size is a 3-inch square

Ingredients

- Slices sourdough bread, 7 slices
- 1/2-inch thick
- Onion, 1 cup
- Raw mushrooms, 1 cup

- Red bell peppers, 1 cup
- Unsalted margarine, 1tbsp
- Fresh spinach leaves, 15
- Large eggs, 7
- Tarragon vinegar, ¼ cup
- Half & half creamer, 1-3/4 cup
- Worcestershire sauce, 1 tsp
- Tabasco® hot sauce, 1 tsp
- Black pepper, 1/2 tsp
- Sharp cheddar cheese, 1 oz. Shredded

Directions

1. Break bread into small squares. Put on the baking tray and for 15 minutes bake at 225° F. Turn them over and bake for 15 minutes more or till crisp and dry.
2. Dice mushrooms, onion, and bell peppers.
3. In a small skillet, Melt margarine and sauté mushrooms, red peppers, and onions.
4. With a cooking spray, grease a baking dish (9-inch square). In the dish, spread half of the bread squares in a single layer and scatter with half of the veggie mixture. Place spinach leaves on this layer.
5. Make a second layer with the remainder bread and veggies on top.
6. Blend together eggs, half & half creamer, vinegar, Worcestershire sauce, black pepper, and hot sauce. Pour over the bread evenly.
7. Keep in the fridge covered with a plastic wrap for about 1 hour or overnight.
8. Bring strata at room temperature by letting stand for 20 minutes outside the fridge.
9. Heat oven to 325° F. Take off the plastic wrap and put it in the oven for 50 minutes.
10. Take out from the oven and scatter cheddar cheese on top. Bake for 10 minutes more or till a

knife comes out clean when inserted near the center

11. Slice into 9 squares and serve hot.

12.

Nutritional Analysis

212 Calories | 12 gr Fat | 11 gr Protein | 15gr Carbohydrates

218 mg Sodium | 347 mg Potassium | 207 mg Phosphorus

60. Fresh Tofu Spring Rolls

Make: 6 Portions

Serving size is 2 spring rolls

Ingredients

- Leaves Romaine lettuce, 12
- Medium carrots, 2
- Medium red onion, 1/2
- Firm tofu, 16 oz
- Ground cumin, 1/2 tbsp
- Granulated garlic, 1/2 tbsp
- Sea salt, 1/4 tsp
- Black pepper, 1/2 tsp
- Olive oil, 1 tbsp
- Rice wrappers, 12 for spring rolls)

Directions

1. Rinse and dry lettuce, then cut each lengthwise in half. Slice the carrots in julienne style. Also, cut the onion. Put aside.

2. To soak the rice wrappers for later, Boil six cups of water and put aside.

3. Rinse and pat dry the tofu. Cut it into 12 slices, about 4 inches long each.

4. Arrange the tofu on a tray and season it with half of the cumin, sea salt, granulated garlic, and black pepper evenly.

5. In a nonstick pan, heat olive oil. Spread the tofu strips in the heated pan, seasoned side down. Sprinkle the Seasoning on the other side and cook until the bottom is slightly browned, for about 1 to 2 minutes. Also, cook the other side till it is also slightly brown. Take out the tofu on a dish to cool.

6. In a shallow, large bowl, pour in the boiled water. Dunk a rice wrapper in that hot water. When it's slightly soft, put the wrapper on a wide plate and arrange 2 pieces of the lettuce in the wrapper's middle. Spoon on top 1- 2 tbsp of sliced onion and 2- 3 tbsp of carrot. Put one cooled strip of tofu on top of the veggies.

7. Bend the sides in, and then folding the bottom up and roll it tightly. Replicate the process with all the rice wrappers, tofu strips, and vegetables.

8. Chill in the fridge and serve cool with your fav dressing, preferably low-sodium.

Nutritional Analysis

156 Calories | 8 gr Protein | 20 gr Carbohydrates | 5 gr Fat

162 mg Sodium | 302 mg Potassium | 93 mg Phosphorus

Stews

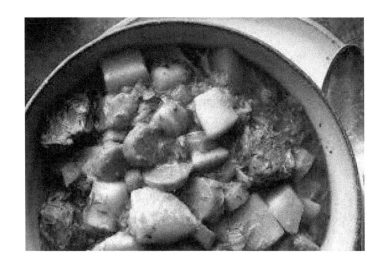

61. Chicken Stew

Makes: 4 portions

Serving size is 1 cup

Ingredients

- Vegetable oil, 3 tbsp
- Chicken breast, 2 pounds, cut into bite-size pieces
- Onions, sliced, 1 cup
- Green peppers, ¾ cup
- Garlic, 2 cloves, minced
- All-purpose flour, 2 tbsp
- Chicken broth, low-sodium, 2 10 ½-oz cans
- Frozen carrots, 1 10-oz bag
- Dried basil, ¼ tsp
- Black pepper, ¼ tsp
- Sliced okra, frozen, 1 110-oz bag

Directions

1. In the Dutch oven, heat 2 tbsp of oil; put in chicken and fry on medium-high heat.

2. Take out chicken and put aside. Add the remainder 1 tbsp of oil.

3. Include and fry the onion, garlic, and pepper.

4. Put in the flour and cook for 2 to 3 minutes, stirring frequently.

5. Add in broth and chicken, cook till starts boiling.

6. Include carrots, black pepper, and basil, simmer covered for around 10 minutes. As it simmers, the gravy will thicken.

7. Cook after adding okra for another 5-10 minutes.

8. Dish up over steaming white rice.

Nutritional Analysis

142 Calories | 10 gr Protein | 8 gr total Fat | 13 gr Carbohydrates

93 mg Sodium | 453 mg Potassium | 129 mg Phosphorus

62. Beef Casserole

Makes: 4 portions

Serving size is ½ cup

Ingredients

- Lean beef, 500g
- Chopped onion, 1 medium
- Carrots, 2, medium, peeled and sliced
- Water, 350ml
- Salt, ¼ tsp
- Vegetable oil, 1 tbsp

- White pepper, ¼ tsp
- Fresh parsley, 1 tbsp, chopped

Directions

1. Fry the chopped onion in the veg oil
2. Put in the beef and sauté until brown
3. Pour in the water and let simmer till beef is almost tender
4. Add in the carrots and cook till meat and carrots are cooked fully.
5. Add in salt and pepper and sprinkle with the freshly chopped parsley.

Nutrition facts

304 Calories | 5 gr Carbohydrate | 21 gr Fat | 23 gr Protein

0.5 gr Sodium | 456 mg Potassium | 202 mg Phosphate

63. Beef Stew with Carrots and Mushrooms

Makes: 8

Serving size is 1 cup.

Ingredients

- White potato, 1 cup
- Onion, 2 cups
- Garlic, 3 cloves
- Carrots, 2 cups
- Beef meat for stew, lean, 2 pounds
- Olive oil, 2 tbsp
- Shitake mushrooms, sliced, 1 cup
- Dried thyme, 1/2 tbsp

- Red wine, 1 cup, dry
- White flour, 1/3 cup, all-purpose
- Herb seasoning blend, 3/4 tsp
- Beef broth, low-sodium, 4 cups
- Bay leaf, 1
- Black pepper, 1/2 tsp

Directions

1. Peel and wash potatoes and make them into small cubes. If on a low potassium diet, double-boil, or soak to decrease potassium.
2. Cut beef into bite-sized pieces. Mince garlic cloves and chop onion. Slice carrots.
3. Heat 2 tsp olive oil in the big Dutch oven on medium-high heat.
4. Put in onions and cook until soft; add in thyme and mushrooms; mix and fry for 5 minutes. Adding garlic sauté for a minute more.
5. To the mixture, add red wine and stir.
6. Dust beef with flour. On medium heat, heat 2 tsp oil in a large frying pan. Add in half of floured beef and season with 1/8 tsp of seasoning blend. Keep cooking until all sides are browned. Repeat the process with the remainder 2 tsp oil, floured beef, and 1/8 tsp seasoning blend.
7. To mushroom mixture, add browned beef.
8. Add bay leaf and broth to mixture. Take to a boil.
9. Decrease the flame to medium-low cover and simmer until beef is tender or for 1 hour.
10. Drain boiled potatoes. Stir in the carrots and potatoes into the pot with beef. Cook on low heat, uncovered for 1 hour, to thicken sauces, stirring occasionally
11. Season with remaining 1/2 tsp seasoning blend and black pepper. Discard bay leaf and serve.

Nutritional Analysis

282 Calories | 33 gr Protein | 10 gr Fat | 15 gr Carbohydrates

110 mg Sodium | 534 mg Potassium | 252 mg Phosphorus

64. Beef Barley Stew

Makes: 6 Portions

Serving size is 1-1/4 cups

Ingredients

- Pearl barley, 1 cup, uncooked
- Onion, 1/2 cup
- Large stalk celery, 1
- Garlic, 1 clove
- Carrots, 2 medium
- Beef stew meat, 1 lb., lean
- White flour, 2 tbsp, all-purpose
- Black pepper, 1/4 tsp
- Canola oil, 2 tbsp
- Bay leaves, 2
- Salt, 1/2 tsp
- Onion herb seasoning, 1 tsp

Directions

1. In 2 cups of water, Soak the barley for 1 hour.
2. Dice the celery and onion. Cut carrots into thick rounds of 1/4-inch each. Grind the garlic clove. Chop the beef into cubes of 1-1/2 inch.
3. Put stew meat, flour, and black pepper in a plastic bag. Vigorously shake to coat beef with

flour.

4. In a 4-quart heavy pot, heat the oil and brown the beef. Take out beef from the pot and put aside.

5. In the meat drippings, Stir and sauté onion, garlic, and celery for 2 minutes. Boil after adding 2 quarts of water. Put back the meat in the pot. Include bay leaves and salt, decrease heat, and let simmer.

6. Rinse and Drain barley, then include in the pot. Cook covered for 1 hour. Stirring every 15 minutes.

7. Add the sliced carrots after 1 hour, season with herb seasoning. Let simmer for 1 more hour. Water can be added to prevent sticking.

Nutritional Analysis

246 Calories | 8 gr Fat | 22 gr Protein | 21 gr Carbohydrates

222 mg Sodium | 369 mg Potassium | 175 mg Phosphorus

65. Chicken and White Bean Chili Stew

Makes: 8 Portions

Serving size is 1 cup

Ingredients

- Chicken breasts, boneless, 1 pound, skinless
- Carrot, ¾ cup
- Black pepper, 1 tsp
- Celery, ¾ cup
- Garlic, 4 cloves
- Onion, ¾ cup
- White beans, 1 cup, canned
- Golden hominy, 15.5 oz. (1 can)

- Chicken broth, 4 cups, low-sodium
- Onions, white pearl, 6, whole
- Green chilies, diced, 4.5 oz canned
- Garlic powder, 2 tsp
- Oregano, 1 tsp
- Ground cumin, 2 tsp
- Cayenne pepper, 1/4 tsp
- Chili powder, 2 tsp

Directions

1. Chop the chicken into small-sized cubes. Sprinkle with black pepper and put in the crock-pot.
2. Dice the celery, carrots, and onion. Finely chop the garlic. To reduce sodium, drain and rinse the beans and hominy.
3. Add the diced onion, carrots, garlic, celery, hominy, beans, pearl onions, chicken broth, and green chilies to the crock-Pot.
4. Add garlic powder, chili powder, cumin, cayenne pepper, and oregano.
5. Cover the lid and cook on low setting for 8 hours in the crock-Pot.

Nutritional Analysis

213 Calories | 5 gr Fat | 19 gr Protein | 23 gr Carbohydrates

354 Sodium | 608 mg Potassium | 232 mg Phosphorus

66. Chicken Pot Pie Stew

Makes: 8 portions

Serving size is 1 cup

Ingredients

- Chicken breast, 1½ pounds, (boneless, skinless)
- Chicken stock, low-sodium 2, cups
- Canola oil, ¼ cup
- Flour, ½ cup
- Fresh carrots, ½ cup, diced
- Fresh onions, ½ cup, diced
- Fresh celery, ¼ cup diced
- Black pepper, ½ tsp
- Italian seasoning, sodium-free, 1 tbsp
- Chicken bouillon, 2 tsp (low sodium)
- Sweet peas, frozen, ½ cup thawed
- Heavy cream, ½ cup
- Piecrust, 1 frozen, cooked, and broken into bite-size pieces
- Cheddar cheese, low-fat, 1 cup

Directions

1. To tenderize pound chicken and chop into small cubes.
2. In a large stockpot, put chicken and stock and for 30 minutes cook on medium-high heat. In the meantime, blend oil and flour until well mixed.
3. Then gradually pour and mix into the chicken broth mixture till it slightly thickens. Decrease heat for 15 minutes to low or medium-low.
4. Add onions, carrots, celery, Italian seasoning, bouillon, and black pepper. Cook for another 15 more minutes.
5. Take off from heat, and then include peas and cream. Mix until combined. Serve in mugs and garnish with same amounts of piecrust and cheese

Nutritional Analysis

388 Calories | 21 gr Total Fat | 22 gr Carbohydrates | 26 gr Protein

424 mg Sodium | 290 mg Phosphorus | 209 mg Potassium

---

67. Kidney-Friendly Navy Bean Stew

Makes: 6 portions

Serving size is 1 cup

Ingredients

- navy Beans, Raw, mature seeds, 1lb, Rinsed thoroughly
- Tomatoes, 2can, packed in tomato juice (15 oz cans), no salt added
- Onion, 1, medium chopped
- Carrots, raw, 1cup grated
- Pepper, 2tbsp
- Seasoned 2.25 Oz
- Taste of Louisiana, 1/2tbsp
- Garlic, 3cloves
- Chicken Bouillon, 2cup, Sodium Free

Directions

1. Immerse 1 lb. navy beans per directions, overnight.
2. Put into a slow cooker with the soaked water.
3. Add in onion, tomatoes, garlic, shredded carrots, Taste of Louisiana Rub, black pepper, and chicken broth.
4. Combine well and simmer for 6-8 hours on low heat.
5. Dish out 1 cup into serving bowl and serve immediately.

6. If any stew is left, it can be kept in the fridge for up to 3 days.

Nutritional Analysis

264 Calories | 1.27 gr Fat | 48.95 Carbohydrates | 16.78 gr Protein

23.44 mg Sodium

Soups

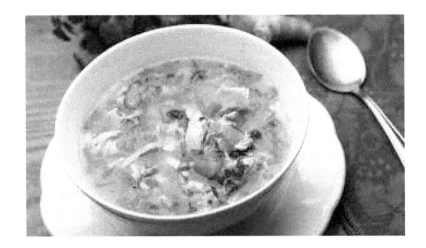

68. Beef & Vegetable Soup

Makes: 8 servings

Serving size is ¾ cup

Ingredients

- Beef stew, 1 pound
- Water, 3 ½ cups
- Sliced onions, 1 cup raw
- Green peas, frozen, ½ cup
- Black pepper, 1 tsp
- Frozen okra, ½ cup
- Basil, ½ tsp
- Carrots, frozen, ½ cup, diced
- Thyme, ½ tsp
- Frozen corn, ½ cup

Directions

1. Place beef stew, black pepper, thyme, onions, basil, and water in a large pot. Cook on medium

for about 45 minutes.

2. Put in all frozen veggies; simmer on decreased heat until meat is soft. Serve hot.

Note: soup can require more water. If necessary, add ½ cup water at a time.

Nutritional Analysis

190 Calories | 11 gr Protein | 13 gr total Fat | 7 gr Carbohydrates

56 mg Sodium | 291 mg Potassium | 121 mg Phosphorus

69. Chicken Noodle Soup

Makes: 8 servings

Serving size is ¾ cup

Ingredients,

- Chicken parts, 1 pound
- Red pepper, 1 tsp
- Lemon juice, ¼ cup
- Caraway seed, 1 tsp
- Water, 3 ½ cups
- Oregano, 1 tsp
- Poultry seasoning, 1 tbsp
- Sugar, 1 tsp
- Garlic powder, 1 tsp
- Celery, ½ cup
- Onion powder, 1 tsp
- Green pepper, ½ cup
- Vegetable oil, 2 tbsp

- Egg noodles, 1 cup
- Black pepper, 1 tsp

Directions

1. Apply lemon juice on chicken parts.
2. Combine chicken, onion powder, garlic powder, poultry seasoning, water in a large pot, also add black pepper, sugar, red pepper, oregano, caraway seed, and vegetable oil together.
3. Cook for 30 minutes or till chicken meat is soft.
4. Add in remaining ingredients and simmer for an added 15 minutes. Dish up hot.

Nutritional Analysis

110 Calories | 8 gr Fat | 3 gr Protein | 7 gr Carbohydrate

17 mg Sodium | 101 mg Potassium | 39 mg Phosphorus

70. Turkey, Wild Rice, and Mushroom Soup

Makes: 6 Portions

Serving size is 1-1/3 cups

Ingredients

- Onion, 1/2 cup
- Bell pepper, red, 1/2 cup
- Carrots, 1/2 cup
- Garlic, 2 cloves
- Turkey, 2 cups, cooked
- Chicken broth, 5 cups, low-sodium
- Wild rice, quick-cooking, 1/2 cup uncooked
- Olive oil, 1 tbsp

- Sliced mushrooms, 4 oz, canned
- Bay leaves, 2
- Herbal seasoning blend, 1/4 tsp
- Dried thyme, 1-1/2 tsp
- Salt, 1/2 tsp
- Black pepper, 1/4 tsp

Directions

1. Chop onion, carrots, and bell pepper. Shred turkey. Mince garlic.
2. In a saucepan, boil 1-3/4 cups broth on medium heat; add in wild rice that is quick-cooking and bring to a boil. Decrease the heat to medium-low. Simmer covered for 5 minutes or till liquid is absorbed. Put aside.
3. In a Dutch oven, heat oil on medium-high heat. Put in bell pepper, onion, garlic, and carrots. Sauté, stirring once in a while.
4. Rinse and drain mushrooms, then add to veggies.
5. Add remainder 3-1/4 cups broth, turkey, bay leaves, thyme, Mrs. Dash seasoning, pepper, and salt to the pan. Cook till it is thoroughly heated, stir.
6. Take out bay leaves and include cooked wild rice in the soup. Serve immediately.

Nutritional Analysis

210 Calories | 5 gr Fat | 23 gr Protein | 15 gr Carbohydrates

270 mg Sodium | 380 mg Potassium | 200 mg Phosphorus

71. Cream of Chicken Wild Rice Asparagus Soup

Makes: 8 portions

Serving size is 3/4 cup for an appetizer portion or 2 cups for a meal.

Ingredients

- Wild rice and long grain blend, 3/4 cups
- Asparagus, 2 cups
- Carrots, 1 cup
- Onion, 1/2 cup
- Garlic, 3 cloves
- Unsalted butter, 1/4 cup
- Thyme, 1/2 tsp
- Pepper, 1/2 tsp, fresh ground
- Nutmeg, 1/4 tsp
- Salt, 1/2 tsp
- Bay leaf, 1
- All-purpose flour, 1/2 cup
- Chicken broth, low-sodium, 4 cups
- Vermouth, extra dry, 1/2 cup
- Cooked chicken, 2 cups
- Almond milk, 4 cups, unsweetened, unenriched

Directions

1. Cook the wild rice blend as per package instructions, quit seasoning packet if given.
2. Take off the pan from flame and let the rice sit, for an added 15 minutes, covered. Put aside and let it cool.
3. Chop the carrots, onion, and asparagus. Finely chop the garlic.
4. Melt the butter in a deep pot, and sauté the onion and garlic until tender. Put in spices, carrots, and herbs. Keep cooking on medium heat until soft.
5. Mixing in the flour, simmer on low heat for around 10 minutes, stirring regularly.

6. Put in all of the vermouth and chicken broth., blend until smooth using a wire whisk.

7. Chop into small pieces the cooked chicken. Add asparagus and chicken to the soup, then gradually add the almond milk. Cook on low heat for 20 minutes.

8. Mix in the prepared wild rice and serve.

Nutritional Analysis

306 Calories | 19 gr Protein | 35 gr Carbohydrates | 10 gr Fat

318 mg Sodium | 475 mg Potassium | 207 mg Phosphorus

72. Spring Vegetable Soup

Makes: 5 Portions

Serving size is 1 cup

Ingredients

- Green beans, 1 cup fresh
- Frozen corn, 1/2 cup
- Celery, 3/4 cup
- Onion, 1/2 cup
- Roma tomato, 1 medium
- Carrots, 1/2 cup
- Olive oil, 2 tbsp
- Mushrooms, 1/2 cup
- Vegetable broth, low-sodium, 4 cups
- Oregano leaves, dried, 1 tsp
- Garlic powder, 1 tsp
- Salt, 1/4 tsp

Directions

1. Remove strings and tips from green beans then cut into pieces of 2-inch. Dice the onion, celery, carrots, tomato, and mushrooms.

2. Heat a large pot on medium flame, add olive oil and lightly fry the onion and celery until soft.

3. Add in the remainder ingredients and bring to a boil. Decrease the heat to make it simmer and cook for around 45 to 60 minutes.

Nutritional Analysis

114 Calories | 6 gr Fat | 2 gr Protein | 13 gr Carbohydrates

262 mg Sodium | 400 mg Potassium | 108 mg Phosphorus

73. Homemade Kidney-Friendly Cream of Mushroom Soup

Makes: 2 portions

Serving size: 1/2 cup

Ingredients

- Unsalted butter, 3 Tbsp
- Onion, finely minced, 1/4 cup
- Mushrooms, finely minced, 1/4 cup
- All-purpose flour, 2 1/2 Tbsp
- Chicken broth, low sodium, 1/2 cup
- Almond milk, unsweetened, 1/2 cup
- Pepper as per taste
- Sea salt as per taste

Directions

1. Take a large skillet of 10", put on medium heat, and melt butter. Put in the onions and cook until soft.

2. Put in mushrooms, cook, and stir for around 5 minutes. Spread flour on veggies and cook for

one minute or two more.

3. Mix in milk and broth and stir till smooth. Cook and bring to a simmer till thick, for about 5 minutes.

Nutritional Analysis

210 Calories | 2.1 gr Protein | 10.2 gr Carbohydrate | 18.2 gr Fat

162.8 mg Sodium | 123.7 mg Potassium | 53.7 mg Phosphorus

74. Rotisserie Chicken Noodle Soup

Makes: 10 Portions

Serving size is 1-1/4 cups

Ingredients

- Rotisserie chicken, prepared, 1
- Chicken broth, low-sodium, 8 cups
- Onion, 1/2 cup
- Celery, 1 cup
- Carrots, 1 cup
- Wide noodles, 6 oz, uncooked
- Fresh parsley, 3 tbsp

Directions

1. Debone the chicken and cut into bite-sized pcs. Take out 4 cups broth for the soup.
2. Into a large stockpot Pour chicken broth; bring to a boil.
3. Dice onion; slice carrots and celery.
4. Add vegetables, noodles, and chicken to the stockpot.
5. Boil it and cook for about 15 minutes till noodles are cooked.
6. Sprinkle chopped parsley on top. Serve

Nutritional Analysis

185 Calories | 5 gr Fat | 21 gr Protein | 14 gr Carbohydrates

361 mg Sodium | 294 mg Potassium | 161 mg Phosphorus

75. Beef and Cabbage Vegetable Soup

Makes: 10 portions

Serving size is 1 cup

Ingredients

- Beef chuck, 1½ pounds chopped
- Water, 10 cups
- Garlic, 1 clove, chopped
- Cabbage, ½ pound, cut into small pieces
- Onion, ½ cup, chopped
- Fresh cilantro, ½ cup, chopped
- Carrots, 2, cut into small pieces
- Tomato sauce, low-salt, ½ cup
- Potato, 1, cut into small pieces
- Stalks celery, 3, cut into small pieces

Directions

1. Simmer in a large pot, meat, garlic, and water for 1 hour.
2. Add all other ingredients and cook on low heat until vegetables are soft.

Nutritional Analysis

26 Calories | 16 gr Fat | 20 gr Protein

Sodium 142 mg, Phosphorus 176 mg, Potassium 413 mg

76. Five Ingredient Vegetable Broth

Makes: 10 portions

Serving size is 1 cup

Ingredients

- Chicken broth, 1 can
- Corn, 1 can, drained and rinsed
- Refried beans, 1 can
- Beans, 1 can, drained and rinsed
- Diced tomatoes, 1 can

All ingredients are fat-free, no salt added, 14.4 oz cans

Directions

1. In a medium pot, combine all ingredients, stirring to mix the refried beans.
2. Cook on low heat, and serve.

Garnish if desired.

Nutritional Analysis

Calories 117 | 21 gr Carbohydrates | 7 gr Protein | 1 gr Fat

378 mg Sodium | 120 mg Phosphorus | 204 mg Potassium 204

77. Hearty Vegetable Soup

Make: 5 portions

Serving size is 1 cup

Ingredients

- Chicken broth, sodium-free, 32 oz. (2 16 oz. Cans)

- Onion, 1 diced
- Carrots, 2 sliced
- Celery stalks, 3 diced
- Green beans, frozen, 2 cups
- White rice, 1 cup (can be replaced with 2 cup noodles)

Directions

1. Chop the onion, celery, and carrots.
2. To a two-quart saucepan, add two cans of salt-free chicken broth and frozen green beans.

For rice

1. Add rice to the pan, cook on low heat till carrots are tender.

For noodles

1. Add noodles after carrots are cooked and cook on low heat till the noodles are soft.

Nutritional Analysis:

105 Calories | 20 gr Carbohydrates | 4 gr Protein | 2 gr Fat

488 mg Sodium

*With rice-

415 mg Potassium | 92 mg Sodium | 96 mg Phosphorus

*With Noodles-

426 mg Potassium | 94 mg Sodium | 125 mg Phosphorus

78. Lower Potassium Potato Soup

Makes: 6 servings

Serving size is 1 cup

Ingredients

- Potatoes, 3, medium
- Low sodium chicken broth, 2 1/4 cups
- Onion, 1/4 cups, chopped
- Celery, 1/2 cups, chopped
- Nondairy creamer, 2 tbsp
- Garlic, 2 small cloves, minced
- Parsley, 1/2 tbsp, dried
- Unsalted butter, 1 1/4 tbsp
- Green onion, 1/2 cups, chopped

Directions

1. In a skillet, heat butter, add onion, garlic, and celery. Cook till tender

2. Add the above to a large saucepan along with broth, demineralized potatoes, non-dairy creamer, and parsley,

3. Keep cooking on low flame for about 20 to 30 minutes

4. Keep stirring and breaking up the potatoes as it simmers. Spoon out into a soup bowl and sprinkle with green onion.

Nutritional Analysis

140 Calories | 4 gr Protein | 21 gr Carbohydrates | 6 gr Fat

52 mg Sodium | 79 mg Phosphorus | 224 mg Potassium

79. Carrot Ginger Soup

Makes: 3 portions

Serving size is 1 cup

Ingredients

- Canola oil, 1/2 tsp

- Carrots, 4. Diced
- Fresh ginger, 2 tbsp, sliced
- Shallot, 1, diced
- Garlic, 1/2 tsp minced
- Horseradish, 1/2 tsp
- Chicken stock, low-sodium, 2 cups
- Tofu, 6 oz, extra firm, silken
- Vinegar, white, 2 tsp
- Sugar, 1 tsp
- Soy sauce, low sodium, 4 drops
- Sesame seed roasted oil, 1/4 tsp

Directions

1. Add oil, ginger, shallots, and carrots to a large saucepan.
2. Cook on medium flame till the carrots seem soft. Add horseradish and garlic, keep cooking for 2 minutes more.
3. Add in chicken stock and crumbled tofu and cook on low heat for 15 minutes. Include sugar, low-salt soy sauce, and vinegar.
4. Puree the soup with a blender. Serve the soup and garnish sesame oil on each bowl.

Nutritional Analysis

129 Calories | 16.5 gr Carbohydrates | 8,4 gr Protein

239 mg Sodium | 112 mg Phosphorus | 566 mg Potassium

Smoothies and Juices

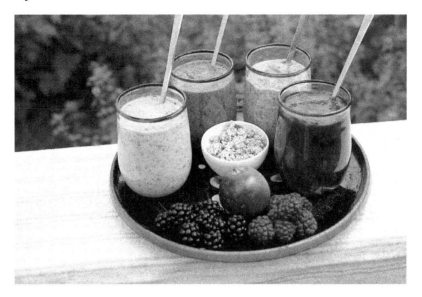

80. Chocolate Smoothie

Makes: 4 portions

Serving size is 6-oz glass

Ingredients

- Whey protein, chocolate-flavored, 2 scoops
- Ice, 2 cups
- Southern comfort liqueur, 2 tbsp, (optional)
- Evaporated milk, ½ cup
- Condensed milk, ¼ cup
- Ground cinnamon, ¼ tsp
- Nutmeg, pinch

Directions

1. In a blender, mix all the ingredients, excluding cinnamon, on high till smooth, approximately for 1 to 2 minutes.
2. Decorate with whipped cream and add a dash of cinnamon to garnish.

Nutritional Analysis

142 Calories | 17 gr Carbohydrates | 10 gr Protein | 4 gr Total Fat

134 mg Sodium | 162 mg Phosphorus | 247 mg Potassium

81. Watermelon Bliss

Makes: 2 portions

Serving size is 1 glass

Ingredients

- Watermelon, 2 cups
- Cucumber, 1 medium, peeled and sliced
- Mint sprigs, 2, leaves only
- Celery stalk, 1
- Squeeze of lime
- Ice cubes

Direction

1. Blend all ingredients in a power blender until smooth.
2. Pour in a tall glass and serve.

Nutritional Analysis

52 Calories | 0 gr Fat | 0 gr Protein | 13 gr Carbohydrates

1 mg Sodium | 9 mg Phosphorus | 96 mg Potassium

82. Cran-tastic

Makes: 1 portion

Serving size is 1 glass

Ingredients

- Frozen cranberries, 1 cup
- Cucumber, 1 medium peeled and sliced
- Celery, 1 stalk
- Squeeze of lime
- A handful of parsley

Direction

1. Put in all ingredients in a blender until smooth.

2. Pour in a tall glass and serve.

Nutritional Analysis

70 Calories | 0.5 gr Fat | 16.5 gr Carbohydrate | 0.3 gr Protein

28.1 mg Sodium | 29.7 mg Potassium | 21.2 mg Phosphorus

83. Bahama Breeze

Makes: 1 portion

Serving size is 1 glass

Ingredients

- Strawberries, ½ cup
- Orange, 1 small, peeled
- Rice milk, ½ cup
- Handful of spinach
- Pineapple, ½ cup
- Ice cubes

Directions

1. Put in all ingredients in a blender until smooth.

2. Pour in a tall glass and serve.

Nutritional Analysis

108 Calories | 27 gr Carbohydrates (5 g with sugar substitute) | 0 gr Fat | 0 gr Protein

2 mg Sodium | 2 mg Phosphorus | 39 mg Potassium

84. Very Berry Goodness

Makes: 1 portion

Serving size is 1 glass

Ingredients

- Cucumber, 1 medium peeled and sliced
- Blueberries, fresh, ½ cup
- Strawberries, fresh or frozen, ½ cup
- Rice milk, ½ cup unsweetened
- Stevia to taste (optional)

Directions

1. Put in all ingredients in a blender until smooth.

2. Pour in a tall glass and serve.

Nutritional Analysis

152 Calories | 4 gr Fat | 14 gr Protein | 15 gr Carbohydrates

84 mg Sodium | 216 mg Potassium | 76 mg Phosphorus

85. What a Peach

Makes: 2 portions

Serving size is 1 glass

Ingredients

- Raspberries, frozen, 1 cup
- Peach, 1 medium pit removed, sliced (or frozen peaches, ½ cup)
- Silken tofu, ½ cup
- Honey, 1 tbsp
- Almond milk, vanilla flavored, unsweetened, 1 cup

Directions

1. Put in all ingredients in a blender until smooth.
2. Pour in a tall glass.

Nutritional Analysis

70 Calories | 0.5 gr Fat | 16.5 gr Carbohydrate | 0.3 gr Protein

28.1 mg Sodium | 29.7 mg Potassium | 21.2 mg Phosphorus

86. Blueberry Blast Smoothie

Makes: 4 Portions

Serving size is 1 cup

Ingredients

- Frozen blueberries, 1 cup
- Splenda, 8 packets
- Protein powder, 6 tbsp
- Ice cubes, 8
- Apple juice, 14 oz (no added sugar)

Directions

1. In a blender, blend all the ingredients and mix until smooth.

Nutritional Analysis

108 Calories | 9 gr Protein | 18 gr Carbohydrates | 0 gr Fat

27 mg Sodium | 183 mg Potassium | 42 mg Phosphorus

87. Easy Pineapple Protein Smoothie

Makes: 1 portion

Serving size is 10 oz

Ingredients

- Pineapple sherbet, 3/4 cup (or sorbet)
- Whey protein powder, vanilla flavor, 1 scoop
- Water, 1/2 cup
- Ice cubes, 2, optional

Direction

1. Add whey protein powder, pineapple sherbet, and water (ice cubes if desired) in a blender.

2. Blend for 30 - 45 seconds; serve immediately.

Nutritional Analysis

268 Calories | 18 gr Protein | 40 gr Carbohydrates | 4 gr Fat

93 mg Sodium | 237 mg Potassium 237 | 160 mg Phosphorus

88. Mixed Berry Protein Smoothie

Makes: 2 portions

Serving size is 7 oz

Ingredients

- Coldwater, 4 oz
- Mixed berries, fresh or frozen, 1 cup
- Ice cubes, 2
- Crystal light, 1 tsp, flavor enhancer drops (liquid, any berry flavor)
- Cream topping, 1/2 cup whipped
- Whey protein, 2 scoops powder

Directions

1. Add frozen berries, ice cubes, water, and crystal light drop in a blender. Blend till mixed well and slushy.

2. Put in protein powder and mix well

3. Put in cream topping and mix well.

4. Makes 2 servings

Nutritional Analysis

152 Calories | 4 gr Fat | 14 gr Protein | 15 gr Carbohydrates

84 mg Sodium | 216 mg Potassium | 76 mg Phosphorus

89. Kidney Nourishing Smoothie

Makes: 2 portions

Serving size is 7 oz

Ingredients

- Cucumber, 1/2 large (peeled and sliced)

- Blueberries, fresh/frozen, 1 cup
- Coconut water, 1 cup (or any nut milk or plain filtered water)
- Chia seeds or ground flax, 1-2 tbsp
- Cinnamon, 1 pinch
- Lime juice, fresh, a good squeeze
- Ice, 1 cup
- Stevia (to taste), optional

Directions

1. In a power blender, add all the ingredients and secure the lid.
2. Turn on the machine and gradually increase the speed to High.
3. Keep scraping the sides of the blender with a spatula if required while processing.
4. Keep Blending for 60 to 90 seconds or till the desired thickness is reached.

Serve and enjoy.

Nutritional Analysis

70 Calories | 0.5 gr Fat | 16.5 gr Carbohydrate | 0.3 gr Protein

28.1 mg Sodium | 29.7 mg Potassium | 21.2 mg Phosphorus

90. Four Ingredient Simple Blueberry Smoothie

Makes: 1

Serving size is 1 glass

Ingredients

- Frozen blueberries, 1/4 cup
- Rice milk, 1 cup
- Honey 1 tsp (or stevia)

- Fresh mint, 1 sprig
- Ice cubes (to obtain desired thickness)

Directions

1. Puree the rice milk, blueberries, honey, extra ice, and mint in a blender. Pour in a tall glass. Serve

Nutritional Analysis

70 Calories | 0.5 gr Fat | 16.5 gr Carbohydrate | 0.3 gr Protein

28.1 mg Sodium | 29.7 mg Potassium | 21.2 mg Phosphorus

91. Watermelon Summer Cooler

Makes: 2 Portions

Serving size is 3/4 cup

Ingredients

- Crushed ice, 1 cup
- Seedless watermelon, 1 cup cubes
- Lime juice, 2 tsp
- Sugar, 1 tbsp
- Watermelon wedges, 2, small for garnish

Directions

1. Blend all the ingredients in a blender, excluding the wedges separated for garnish, and blend well for 30 seconds.
2. Take out into two medium glasses, garnish with wedges and serve!

Nutritional Analysis:

52 Calories | 13 gr Carbohydrates | 0 gr Protein | 0 gr Fat

1 mg Sodium | 9 mg Phosphorus | 96 mg Potassium

92. Lemonade

Makes: 10 portions

Serving size is 3 oz water + 3 oz base

Ingredients

- Water, 2-1/2 cups
- Sugar, 1-1/4 cups (or sugar substitute)
- Lemon, finely shredded, 1/2 tsp (or lime peel)
- Lemon, fresh, 1-1/4 cups (or lime juice)
- Ice cubes

Directions

1. Mix the water and sugar substitute or sugar in a medium saucepan, on medium heat till the sugar is dissolved. Take off from the heat and cool for 20 minutes.
2. Put in the juice and citrus peel to the sugar mix. Pour out into a pitcher or a jar; chill covered. It can be kept for up to 3 days.
3. To make a glass of lemonade, mix base 3 oz and water 3 oz in a glass filled with ice. Stir and enjoy it. The leftover base can be frozen in ice trays and used as ice in drinks.

Nutritional Analysis:

108 Calories | 0 gr Fat | 0 gr Protein | 27 gr Carbohydrates (5 g with sugar substitute)

2 mg Sodium | 2 mg Phosphorus | 39 mg Potassium

Desserts

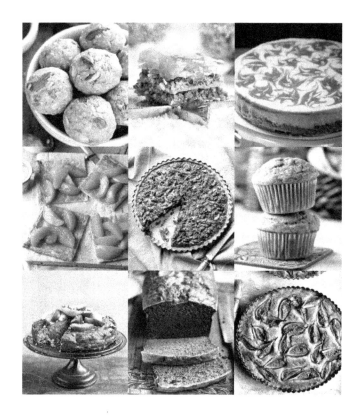

93. Scarlet Frozen Fantasy

Makes: 4 portions

Serving size is 4 oz

Ingredients

- Cranberry, 1 cup, juice cocktail
- Strawberries, fresh, whole, 1 cup, washed and hulled
- Lime juice, 2 tbsp, fresh
- Sugar, ¼ cup
- Ice cubes, 8-9
- For garnish: strawberries

Directions

1. Combine strawberries, cranberry juice, sugar, and lime juice in a blender. Blend well.

2. Adding ice cubes again. Mix until smooth.

3. Serve in chilled glasses. Decorate it with a strawberry.

Nutritional Analysis

100 Calories | 0 gr Protein | 0 gr total Fat | 24 gr Carbohydrate

3 mg Sodium | 109 mg Potassium | 129 mg Phosphorus

94. Baked Egg Custard

Makes: 4 portions

Serving size is ½ cup

Ingredients

- Eggs, 2, medium
- 2% milk, ¼ cup
- Sugar, 3 tbsp
- Vanilla, 1 tsp (or lemon extract)
- Nutmeg, 1 tsp

Directions

1. Heat oven to 325°F.
2. Bring together all ingredients and with an electric mixture, beat for a minute until well mixed.
3. spoon into muffin pans or custard cups.
4. Sprinkle nutmeg on each.
5. Bake for at least 20 to 30 minutes or till a knife inserted in the custard comes out clean.

Nutritional Analysis

70 Calories | 3 gr Protein | 9 gr Carbohydrate | 3 gr Fat

34 mg Sodium | 30 mg Potassium | 42 mg Phosphorus

95. Pineapple Pudding

Makes: 12 portions

Serving size is ½ cup

Ingredients

- All-purpose flour, 3 tbsp
- Sugar, ½ cup
- Egg, 1 large, whole
- Eggs, 3, large, divided
- 2% milk, 1 cup
- Water, 1 cup
- Vanilla extract, 1 tsp
- Pineapple chunks, 2 cups, drained
- Sugar, ¼ cup
- Vanilla wafers, 25-30

Directions

1. Heat oven to 425°F.
2. Combine 3 egg yolks, 1 whole egg, flour and, sugar in a double boiler.
3. Stir in water and milk. Cook, over boiling water, uncovered, stirring continually, until thickened.
4. Take off from heat, and include vanilla extract.
5. In a casserole dish of 1 ½ quart, spread a small quantity of custard; arrange half of the vanilla wafers and then half of the pineapple over it.
6. Continue layering custard, pineapple, and vanilla wafers, beginning and finishing with custard.

7. Beat the remainder egg whites with a hand mixer or egg beater, add sugar. Beat till hard peaks form.

8. Spoon stiff egg whites on the layered pudding. Bake until lightly brown or for 5 minutes.

Nutritional Analysis

209 Calories | 4 gr Protein | 5 gr total Fat | 38 gr Carbohydrate

80 mg Sodium | 120 mg Potassium | 71 mg Phosphorus

96. Old Fashioned Pound Cake

Makes: 24 portions

Serving size is 1 slice

Ingredients

- Eggs, 6
- Butter, 2 cups
- Powdered sugar, 4 cups
- All-purpose flour, 3 ½ cups, sifted
- Lemon rind, grated, 2 tbsps.
- Lemon extract, 1 tsp

Directions

1. Heat oven to 350°F.
2. with an electric mixer, for 3 minutes cream butter on medium speed till fluffy and light.
3. Slowly add sugar and le3mon rind; beat thoroughly.
4. Add in the extract of lemon and eggs, one at a time, blending well after each adding.
5. Slowly add flour; mix thoroughly.
6. grease and flour a 10" Bundt pan or tube pan and pour the mixture in.

7. Bake for almost one hour and twenty minutes or till a wooden pick comes out clean when put in in the center.
8. Remove from oven and cool.

Nutritional Analysis

279 Calories | 10 gr Protein | 34 gr Carbohydrate

127 mg Sodium | 108 mg Potassium | 139 mg Phosphorus

97. Carrot Cake

Makes: 15 squares

Serving size is 1 square (3" x 6")

Ingredients for cake

- Granulated sugar, 1 cup
- Vegetable oil, ½ cup
- Eggs, 2
- Carrots, 1 ½ cup, grated or shredded
- Vanilla extract, 1 tsp
- All-purpose flour, 2 cups
- Nutmeg, ¼ tsp
- Baking soda, 2 tsp
- Baking powder, 1 tsp
- Ground cinnamon, 2 tsp
- Ground cloves, ¼ tsp
- Pineapples, canned, 1 cup crushed

Directions for cake

1. Heat oven to 375°F.

2. Mix egg, oil, and sugar; beat well.

3. Put in vanilla and carrots. Beat till smooth mixture forms.

4. Add the remainder ingredients to the mixture and mix well.

5. Grease and flour a 9" x 13" cake pan, pour the mixture in it.

6. Bake for at least 30 minutes. Cool for 10 minutes. Take out from the pan.

7. top with icing or Garnish with whipped cream (optional).

Ingredients for icing

- Cream cheese, 1 bar, softened, 4-oz
- Unsalted margarine, ¼ cup softened
- Vanilla, 1 tbsp
- Powdered sugar, 2 cups, sifted

Directions for icing

1. Beat together unsalted margarine and cream cheese. Add in powdered sugar and vanilla.

2. Layer over cool cake. (extra powdered sugar Maybe needed to harden the icing).

Nutritional Analysis

202 Calories | 3 gr Protein | 8 gr total Fat | 30 gr Carbohydrates

94 mg Sodium | 81 mg Potassium | 44 mg Phosphorus

98. Pumpkin Strudel

Makes: 8 portions

Serving size is 1 slice

Ingredients

- Unsweetened pumpkin, 1½ cups canned, sodium-free,
- Grated nutmeg, ⅛ tsp

- Vanilla extract, 1 tsp
- Sugar, 4 tbsp
- Ground cinnamon, ½ tsp
- Butter, unsalted, 4 tbsp, (½ stick), melted
- Phyllo dough, 12 sheets (if frozen, follow package instructions for defrosting)

Directions

1. Preheat the oven to 380° F. Arrange the oven rack in the center of the oven.
2. In a medium-sized mixing bowl, mix the canned pumpkin, vanilla extract, nutmeg, ½ tbsp of cinnamon, and 2 tbsp of sugar until well-mixed.
3. With a pastry brush, coat a nonstick medium baking tray with butter. Lay flat a single phyllo dough sheet on a clean work table, and apply butter to it. Then stack buttered phyllo sheets one by one on, brushing each phyllo sheet with melted butter. (Do save a little quantity of melted butter for brushing the top of strudel.) Keep covered remaining phyllo sheets with plastic wrap till ready for use.
4. Spread the mixture along one of the stack's longer sides evenly when all 12 sheets are done. Begin to roll from the filling end to the empty end; make sure the seam-side is downwards.
5. On the greased sheet tray, transfer the roll seam-side downward and brush with the remainder butter.
6. Mix the remaining cinnamon and sugar in a small bowl. Spread it on the sides and top of the strudel.
7. Place on the oven's center rack until golden brown or lightly toasted, about 12 to 15 minutes.
8. Take out the baked strudel from the oven and let the toasted strudel rest for about 5 to 10 minutes.
9. Let the center settle, then Slice with a sharp knife and Serve.

Nutritional Analysis

180 Calories | 8 gr total Fat | 25 gr Carbohydrates | 3 gr Protein

141 mg Sodium | 39 mg Phosphorus | 119 mg Potassium

99. Sunburst Lemon Bars

Makes: 24 bars

Serving size is 1 bar

Ingredients

Crust:

- All-purpose flour, 2 cups
- Powdered sugar, ½ cup
- Butter, unsalted, 1 cup (2 sticks), room temperature

Filling:

- Eggs, 4
- Sugar, 1½ cups
- All-purpose flour, ¼ cup
- Cream of tartar, ½ tsp
- Baking soda, ¼ tsp
- Lemon juice, ¼ cup

Glaze:

- Powdered sugar, 1 cup, sifted
- Lemon juice, 2 tbsp

Directions

Crust:

1. Heat oven to 350° F.
2. Combine the flour, 1 cup of softened butter, and powdered sugar in a large bowl. Combine

until crumbly. In a 9" x 13" baking pan, flatten the mixture into the bottom.

3. Bake for about 15 to 20 minutes until lightly browned.

Filling:

1. Whisk the eggs lightly in a medium mixing bowl.

2. Take another bowl, mix the flour, sugar, baking soda, and cream of tartar. Mix the dry mixture in the eggs. Also, add the lemon juice and beat until it gets slightly thick.

3. Pour the mix on the warm crust and then bake for 20 minutes more or till filling is set.

4. Take out and put aside to cool.

Glaze:

1. Take a small bowl, slowly stir the juice of a lemon into the powdered sugar that is sifted, until spreadable. Put more or less juice of the lemon as desired.

2. Spread glaze on the cooled filling. Set aside to set the glaze and then slice into 24 bars. Extra lemon bars be stored in the refrigerator.

Nutritional Analysis

200 Calories | 9 gr Total Fat | 28 gr Carbohydrates | 2 gr Protein

27 mg Sodium | 32 mg Phosphorus | 41 mg Potassium

100. Fruit in The Clouds

Makes: 4 squares

Serving size is 1 square of 2" x 2"

Ingredients

- Fruit cocktail, 1 can, drained
- Mandarin orange, 1 can, drained
- Whipped cream, 8 oz frozen

Directions

1. Combine all ingredients together.
2. Pour in individual molds or 8" x 8" container. Freeze.

Nutritional Analysis

113 Calories | 1 gr Protein | 3 gr total Fat | 23 gr Carbohydrates

20 mg Sodium | 152 mg Potassium | 29 mg Phosphorus

Conclusion

Kidney disease needs a systematic approach to decrease symptoms and enhance the patient's quality of life. In the treatment of kidney failure, food patterns play a critical role. Therefore, to manage the disease and avoid dialysis, the most effective thing you can do is follow a renal diet.

To decrease the volume of waste in their blood, individuals with kidney disease must stick to a renal diet. Blood waste occurs from food and drinks that are ingested. As kidney activity is affected, the kidneys do not adequately filter or extract waste. It will adversely influence the electrolyte levels of a patient if an excess is left in the blood. Following a renal diet could also help improve kidney functionality and delay the progression of chronic kidney disease.

The renal diet is low in phosphorous, protein, and sodium. This diet emphasizes the importance of eating good protein and limiting liquids. Calcium and potassium will also need to be restricted in certain patients. Every individual's body is different, so each patient needs to collaborate with a renal dietitian to create a diet customized to the needs of the patient.

For patients with CKD at all levels, an adequate diet is important. Numerous reports suggest that diets high in fruits, cereals, vegetables, seafood, fibers, whole grains, and polyunsaturated fatty acids but poor in saturated fatty acids are necessary for people with CKD. A low protein diet fortified with ketoacids (s-VLPD) and amino acids was also shown to be healthy and helpful for people with CKD, particularly at stages 4 and 5, since it corrects hemoglobin, blood pressure, and proteinuria, and can therefore extend not only the dialysis-free duration but also the patient's life.

CPSIA information can be obtained
at www.ICGtesting.com
Printed in the USA
LVHW050719301120
672997LV00001B/43